Vegetarian Ketogenic Diet

*Combining and Understanding
a Vegetarian and Keto - Diet Lifestyle*

+

Easy recipes Ideas

+

*Bonus 7 Days Meal Plans, Lose Weight and
Feel More Energetic for Beginners and Not*

Tim Martin

no scenarios in which the publisher or the original author of this work can be in any fashion deemed liable for any hardship or damages that may befall them after undertaking information described herein.

Additionally, the information in the following pages is intended only for informational purposes and should thus be thought of as universal. As befitting its nature, it is presented without assurance regarding its prolonged validity or interim quality. Trademarks that are mentioned are done without written consent and can in no way be considered an endorsement from the trademark holder.

Table of Contents

Chapter 1

What a Vegetarian Diet Is and How It Works to Benefit Your Health and the Health of the Planet

If you've ever wanted to lose weight, you have probably asked yourself which diet is the best for you and what diet will make the best and healthiest version of yourself. For thousands of people, the answer is simple—vegetarianism. As with any diet you choose, you should consult your doctor and find out if it is safe for you. In this book, we are going to give you vital information about this diet to help give you more information as well. In countries all over the world, vegetarianism is on the rise. Some countries have hundreds in just one city. People adopt a vegetarian lifestyle for many reasons. Some believe that animals should not be eaten or harmed for our food and that humans are selfish for using them in our daily lives. Others argue that we should not use animal products at all because they believe that we should leave animals alone and that they should live their natural life in peace. Others have religious beliefs that express that they cannot partake of meat. Others still may have cultural beliefs as to why they cannot eat meat.

Meanwhile, some may just want to get healthy and fit to extend their lives even just a bit.

Whatever the reasoning behind it, the vegetarian diet is definitely something that is worth looking into. There are also many different types of vegetarians out there, but the basic definition of a vegetarian is someone who abstains from eating meat—but unlike vegans, they might still eat eggs, milk, and other dairy products or still use animal products in their daily life. For example, a vegan would never wear leather or fur because they think it is morally wrong to wear a part of an animal. A vegetarian might not have the same problem and own a fur coat or leather coat and wear it often. Another example is a vegan would never consume honey. Most vegetarians do because they think it is a tasty addition to their diet. Unfortunately for you, honey is a no-go on a ketogenic diet—it has way too many carbs. To break down the different types of vegetarianism so that you can choose which would suit your needs and desires along with the goals you have set for yourself, we will define the other types of vegetarianism as well.

A **lacto vegetarian** is a person who does not eat meat or eggs, but they consume other dairy products such as cheese, milk, yogurt, or ice cream.

A **lacto ovo vegetarian** is someone who avoids meat but does consume eggs and other types of dairy products like the ones listed above.

Ovo vegetarians avoid all animal products except

eggs—meaning that they do not eat meat or dairy at all except for eggs.

Adopting the vegetarian lifestyle is quite a switch if you are used to eating a lot of meat, and finding the right diet may seem hard—but one thing all of these diets have in common is that they will not consume any animal flesh whatsoever. After that, you can go from there and decide how far you would like to take your personal vegetarianism. Some like to remain as they are, while there are some that may decide to take it further and end up becoming a vegan, which is a more restrictive diet than vegetarianism or ketogenic diet.

One of the things that people love about vegetarianism is that it is beneficial not just to you but to the planet as well. A word of caution, though, would be to eat wisely. Think for a second—you are adopting a vegetarian diet for your health, right? There may be other reasons as well, but you are at least partially doing this to feel better. This means being careful about what you put in your body. A good example is the fact that chocolate cake, fudge brownies, and ice cream sundaes are all vegetarian. Pies, chips from the store, and candy bars are also all vegetarian. However, they are not really that good for you. In fact, they are not the least bit healthy at all. Hence, you really need to observe your habits and to be sure about changing them. Also, as a vegetarian, you can still gain weight. Even if you eat healthy foods, you need to control your portions and make sure you are not overeating. With a vegetarian diet, you are eating more vegetables and things of the nature, so it is actually pretty easy to overeat because you cannot tell sometimes that you are, as it does not seem that way. Even overeating on plant-based foods can make your weight fluctuate or begin to rise even if you were trying to achieve the opposite. Another example is fake meat and fake cheese—these are obviously mere substitutes for the real thing. Some are amazing for the ketogenic diet; others are packed full of calories, fat, and carbs. On this particular diet, you have to remember to keep the carbs low. You only get five percent—that's it! If you go over, you bust your budget. They may also be full of trans fat and processed sugar. Processed sugar is also something that we are avoiding here. This is going to make you gain weight and can cause issues that you do not want in your diet.

There have been many sites and books written about the health benefits and risks of a vegetarian diet—and the first thing that many sites agree on is that there is not enough evidence to show long-term benefits because everyone is different, and you may live your life totally opposite of how someone else does. For example, I am not a drinker. Alcohol and beer are, of course, vegetarian, as there is no meat. Hence, if you are a vegetarian that drinks and I am not, or if I am a vegetarian that does not drink and also works out every day but you are not—you obviously are going to have health issues that I do not. Another example is you are a vegetarian that smokes you will have health issues that others do not. Alternatively, if someone is a vegetarian but they live in a city or country that is being exposed to unhealthy things (which, unfortunately, many countries across the globe are), their health is going to be vastly different as well because your country may not be being exposed to the same things. Also, if someone is obese, they will have health problems that someone who has a healthy weight will not because obesity can cause many different health issues.

That being said, there are some things that researchers agree on. Most agree that meat eaters weigh more than vegetarians and that maintaining a healthier weight is a great benefit to eating a plant-based diet instead of a meat diet. This is probably because you are cutting out the hormones and possibly cancer-causing problems that can arise from you eating meat. If you are a man, another benefit of cutting out meat from your diet is that studies and certain evidence have shown that meat can actually cause erectile dysfunction over prolonged eating. Sounds crazy, right? However, the foods you eat can actually have a really big effect on your body and mind.

Another great health benefit of vegetarianism is that if you have high blood pressure or even hypertension, which can be a very scary thing to deal with, studies have shown that because a lot of vegetarians are able to maintain a healthy weight it can lower these symptoms and could leave you feeling healthier and lead to more energy which could end up helping you free yourself of these problems. Hypertension has four stages and each one gets progressively worse. Stage one is known as prehypertension, stage two is mild hypertension, stage three is moderate hypertension and finally, stage four is severe hypertension. Hypertension occurs when you have a persistent abnormal elevation of the pressure that's within the arteries. The arteries deliver blood to the entire body. High blood pressure needs to be taken very seriously if you have it because it can lead to stroke, blindness, kidney failure or fatal effects like heart failure or a heart attack.

Heart disease is also something that can be scary to think about. A vegetarian diet has a lot of unsaturated fats. Examples of unsaturated fats for vegetarians would be avocados, nuts, soybeans, seeds, and olives. Plant-based foods have been researched and some studies have said that they tend to reduce the risk of heart disease and they are less likely to develop ischemic heart disease.

A study that was done about five years ago, studied more than seventy thousand people. They discovered that vegetarians had had a twelve percent lower risk of death. This was compared with the non-vegetarians.

Another study that was done a little further back showed when they split people randomly on three diets, one vegetarian no meat, one all meat allowed, and one only fish only, after two weeks the vegetarians had mood improvements. More so than the other two diets.

Vegetarianism is said to be a great benefit for our planet as well, although there is much speculation regarding this. One of the benefits of going vegetarian is said to be the reduction of our ecological footprint. It is said that by going plant-based we reduce the water, oil and land resources that meat and animal products make us use more of. It can also cut back on the amount of pollution we produce as well as saving more than one hundred animals each year by not consuming their flesh.

Deforestation is another big problem in today's society and it is widely believed that the livestock industry is the cause. Many industries tell us that if we were to even cut down on our meat the livestock industry would not be able to cause so much damage and animals would not have to be without their homes.

There has been the saying that water is not an infinite resource and the earth does not have enough for ages. The information varies from source to source but the guesswork of how much water it takes to produce just one kilo of beef can vary from thirteen thousand liters to even one hundred thousand liters. Clearly, that's a massive amount of water being used for just one kilo. Imagine how much water is being used for a cities supply of meat—or an entire continent. To take your perception even further, it only takes one thousand to two thousand liters to produce one kilo of wheat. That's a far cry from the thirteen thousand it takes for beef is not it?

We've all heard of global warming, right? The vice president has mentioned it, celebrities have mentioned it, it is everywhere you look. Many children learn in school about the damage to the ozone layer and celebrate Earth Day and try to be clean and help the planet. Many people have theorized that animals produce more greenhouse gases than all of the cars on the planet. That's' a lot of gas. They further theorize that by adopting a vegetarian diet and not eating the animals you can vastly reduce the number of greenhouse gases and save the planet from getting hurt more than it already is. While people are discovering if we can reverse the damage it has been told to us that we can try and stop the planet from getting worse.

Along with greenhouse gases, sheep and cows make up about thirty-seven percent of the methane that is being emitted into our air. These statistics for methane are twenty-three times as warming as the co2 that's being emitted. Thirty-seven percent is nearly half of the methane emissions. That's a completely insane amount of emissions. We need to reduce this number as much as possible and quickly. Acid rain is being contributed to as well by ammonia emissions which thanks to the livestock industry is said to be sixty-four percent. Manure from the animals was consuming produces sixty-five percent of nitrous oxide that's human-related or caused. That is about three hundred times the global warming potential of Co2 that's produced. A vegetarian diet can cut these numbers down as well and begin to reduce emissions simply from taking the meat out of your diet.

Since vegetarians are not consuming meat and the animal protein that comes with it, especially processed meat or red meat, your chances of getting type two diabetes goes down as well. Even omnivores, who of course eat both plant-based foods and meats, who consumed meat even once a week or more of a prolonged period of time had a seventy-four percent higher risk of catching this horrible disease.

Our human population keeps getting bigger and it is expected that it will grow by three billion. It is also said that there will be plans to help poorer countries get more meat to feed their people, which means that in the next few decades, we will need more animals to eat. Many people believe that this is going to be a massive food crisis later on. Also, it has been said that because vegetarians survive mostly on vegetables and not meat, they need less living space. Meaning that they could survive on less land than those who survive mostly on meat. A good example of this would be that a family that lives in Bangladesh, living off of just rice, vegetables, and other vegetarian items would need less land and farming because they would not be raising cattle or pigs or the other animals that carnivores or omnivores consume daily. But the average family that lives in America can consume around two hundred and seventy pounds of meat in just a year. So they would need twenty times as much land.

It is said that about thirty percent of the available surface of the planet that is ice-free, is being used by livestock. Unfortunately, there are one billion people who cannot eat and go hungry every day and livestock consume most of the world's crops. Another downside is that our hunger for meat has led to desertification and soil erosion and it puts so much extra stress on people's homelands. Overgrazing from the uplands of Ethiopia to the mountains of Nepal or the downlands of southern England also causes flooding and great losses of fertility.

Another thing to think about is in some farms where they raise cattle for meat, they are ensured to be raised in a way that packs the most meat on them as they possibly can before they are killed for us. This is not true in countries that are not as well off. The cattle in poorer countries is essential for some people's way of life. It ensures they have a job and food. Without it, they would not.

There is also so much water used to raise animals. Studies have shown it takes about nine thousand liters of water or in pounds that's twenty thousand, to produce one pound of beef. Additionally, to produce one liter of milk, nearly one thousand liters of water are needed. Or a broiler chicken takes much less than beef, but it still needs one thousand five hundred liters of water. Another example of how much water is used is pigs. Pigs are said to be some of the thirstiest animals. If you are looking at it, his way an average sized pig farm in North America will have about eighty thousand pigs. Those eighty thousand pigs need nearly seventy-five million gallons much needed water over the course of a single year. That number grows exponentially when you think of the size of the farms in bigger cities. If you think about that for a second that is a lot of water that could be used for other things. As a vegetarian, you will have the knowledge that you are not contributing to those numbers. You will be saving so much water simply by not eating any of the meat that uses so much of our water.

Richer countries that are water stressed such as South Africa, and Libya or Saudi Arabia say that it makes sense that poorer countries grow food to conserve their water resources. Some countries are even trying to help others buy growing their cows in their countries then sending them to others.

We could be poisoning the earth. When animals excrete manure and you have hundreds or thousands in a tiny area the manure is funneled along with the urine into a waste lagoon that can hold massive amounts. Some hold as much as forty million gallons. The cesspools often break and leak or overflow because they are holding so much, and this pollutes water supplies and underground water supplies as well. It also pollutes rivers with phosphorus and nitrates along with nitrogen. There are thousands of miles of rivers in Europe, Asia, and the United States that are polluted each and every year.

The sheer number of animals that people need or choose to eat is harming the earth in other ways as well. We could be hurting our planet's biodiversity. The definition of biodiversity tells us that it is the variety of life in a particular habitat or in the world or a particular ecosystem. The reason that biodiversity is important is that it boosts productivity in an ecosystem where all species no matter how big or small all have a part to play. An example to help you understand would be if you imagine a large number of plant life or species. Larger plant life equals a larger variety of crops. If we have greater species diversity, we are ensuring sustainability for all life forms. But not just sustainability. Natural sustainability.

We are spoiling the oceans of the world and killing innocent sea life. When so much excess waste gets dumped into the water the fish begin to die for no reason other than humans are polluting the only home they have.

There are nearly four hundred dead zones and they range in all different sizes. They've ranged from one square kilometer to over seventy thousand square kilometers. They've been identified from the South China Sea to the Scandinavian fjords. The culprit of these dead zones is not only animal farming, but it is one of the worst as it causes so much damage.

Animal waste is making us more prone to getting sick because many of the pathogens in animal waste include E coli, bacteria that can be transferred so easily hundreds could get infected and cryptosporidium. Cryptosporidium is what is a genus of apicomplexan parasitic alveolate. It can cause a gastrointestinal illness or respiratory illness. The main problem this causes is watery diarrhea and it comes with or without a cough. If you do get this cough it will be pretty persistent. In addition, another problem with livestock is that they do not grow fast enough or have enough meat for the farmers and each year they need more and more meat. So they have to resort to new methods. Those methods for getting them to produce more, also have an effect on us and how we get sick.

Another bad thing about eating meat? The quantity of meat that people consume is absolutely staggering. Studies over time have shown that on average a British carnivore will eat about or even over eleven thousand animals in their lifetime. These animals include twenty-eight ducks, one thousand one hundred and fifty-eight chickens, three thousand five hundred ninety-three shellfish, four cattle, six thousand one hundred and eighty-two fish, eighteen pigs, thirty-nine turkeys, one rabbit, twenty-three lambs and sheep, and one goose.

The vegetarians are speaking up about this saying that because of this, the meat eaters have increased chances of becoming obese. They also say that heart disease and cancer can come from this as well.

There are so many problems with this world because the meat was consuming many of them listed above. In your life as a vegetarian, you can save hundreds of animals from the fate of being hurt and you can begin to help the planet from these horrible issues that have been arising from livestock. A vegetarian does benefit everyone because you are not contributing to the production of these animal farms, which are hurting the planet and the people who inhabit it.

Chapter 2

What a Ketogenic Diet Is and How and Why It Can Improve Your Health

When adopting a vegetarian diet, you might also decide you want to adopt the ketogenic diet and combine that with your food choices. A ketogenic diet is a diet that focuses on being very low in carbs and very high in fats. It can share certain similarities with other well-known low-carb diets. What this diet is designed to do is put your body into a state called *ketosis*. This is a metabolic state that is a reduction of carbs, and it means you are reducing how much you gain carbs and instead replacing them with fats. They believe that when you adopt this diet, your body will become more efficient at burning your fat and turning it into energy. It also believes that the fats in your liver will turn into ketones. After they turn to ketones, it is said by some that your brain will now have more energy because of this process.

As with a vegetarian diet, there are people who classify themselves as a different type of ketogenic. While there is a debate on which is the best, there are four that are most commonly chosen among people.

The high protein ketogenic diet, which has things in common with a standard ketogenic diet but as the title implies, this diet has more protein than the standard version. The ratio is, of course, different as well. For a high protein ketogenic diet, you have thirty-five percent protein, with sixty percent fat and only five percent is made up of carbs.

A cyclical ketogenic diet is a diet that uses the idea of refeeding. Refeeding is the process of eating more calories than you have in previous days. People believe that the process of refeeding is beneficial in losing fat because it is supposed to boost metabolism and ideally stop you from falling into a calorie deficit or crashing. So, this diet will be using higher refeeds than the other forms of ketogenic diets on this list. This is the only one on this list that allows you to have 'cheat days. They believe you should have two higher carb days and five ketogenic days. They also stress that the two carb days should follow the ketogenic days and not before.

The targeted ketogenic diet is the simplest diet on this list because the only difference it has to the other diets is that this diet believes it is beneficial to add carbs around your workouts.

Finally, we come to the standard ketogenic diet. This is the most popular of the four and most people choose this diet as their go-to for this lifestyle. The standard diet believes that you should have only twenty percent protein and five percent carbs but have a seventy-five percent allowance for your fat. It is most assuredly a high-fat diet with extremely low carbs but still maintaining moderate protein. The thing to remember here is low carb. There are many vegetarian foods that you should not eat on a ketogenic diet like pasta, tortillas, bread, pretzels and other snack foods like chips or crackers, soda, cereal, fruit juices, and most fruits. These are all too high in carbs for a ketogenic diet. You'll need to stay away from packaged foods with refined flour or sugar, rice, white potatoes, and sweet potatoes and starchy vegetables. There are still plenty of other items you can eat so if it seems like you are really limited, you are not. You just need to work around what you cannot eat.

Any of these diets would benefit your help although obviously as each diet has differences, you will need to determine which is going to help you the most because you know what your goals are.

Originally a ketogenic diet was believed to be a helpful aid to help with epilepsy and seizures. One of the things that are stressed about this is that since the ketogenic diet is very specialized it needs to be done with the guidance, supervision, and care of trained medical specialists. In certain countries of the world, they will only offer adult treatment in very few clinics because more data and research are needed about the impact the diet will have on adults. Through careful monitoring with specialists, doctors, and nutritionists, they say that there can be benefits for children with epilepsy and seizures using this diet, but they are still conducting more research on this as well.

Other studies have shown that the ketogenic diet may

reduce symptoms of Parkinson's disease or polycystic ovary syndrome in women by reducing insulin levels. It has been debated in others that it may be used to treat different kinds of cancer or tumor growth or reduce symptoms of Alzheimer's disease or possibly slow down its progression. When scientists did a study on animals, they learned that on an animal brain the diet could reduce concussions and help recovery after a brain injury—but obviously, an animal's brain is vastly different than humans, and we do not know if the same results would be reflected in a human brain.

It has been debated in certain cases, but it some cases people found that some of the test subjects lost two times more weight on the ketogenic diet than on a low-fat diet that restricts calories. Like veganism, which means that you do not consume any animal product at all whatsoever, a ketogenic diet is also said to help with type two diabetes, but the ketogenic diet is said in one study to have improved insulin by seventy-five percent.

Another study even found that in the study they performed, seven people out of the twenty-one participants were able to stop using their diabetic medication. Now obviously that does not mean it will happen for everyone as everyone's health and body can be different and some people may have had diabetes longer than others. That's why more research is needed on the subject so that we can get more concrete answers and evidence.

Chapter 3

The Dangers That Can Arise from a Vegetarian Ketogenic Diet

There are dangers that can be found in any diet you choose—and unfortunately, there is a set of dangers with this diet as well, and they should be mentioned because it would not be to your benefit if we only mentioned the positives without informing you of the possible side effects that can happen and the effects it can have on your body. Because you are combining two diets into one here, unfortunately, that means you can have twice the dangers than other diets. The vegetarian ketogenic diet can also have damaging effects on the planet as well—which sounds quite crazy—but is true.

Most people say that they become vegetarians to help the planet, so most find it incredible that a vegetarian diet might actually hurt the planet. Recent studies, however, show that a diet with more fruits and vegetables and less meat might actually exact a higher environmental toll than the way we eat now. According to some recent findings, shifting our diets would increase energy use by up to thirty-eight percent, and it would increase greenhouse gas

23

emissions by up to six percent and water use by up to ten percent.

As everyone knows greenhouse gas emissions are causing so many problems to our planet and air. Scientists and environmentally minded activists everywhere are trying to lower these greenhouse gasses and come up with a solution, which is why so many people lean toward a plant-based diet. They are trying to reduce their carbon footprint and the damage we do to the planet. The shocking thing though is that if you are going by calories, making Lettuce can create as much greenhouse emissions as beef. It has been shown that lettuce generates about three times what pork or fresh fish. For vegetarians they eat more green vegetables, so they would most likely turn to lettuce in their diet—meaning, they would be inadvertently doing something that might not be helpful even though they did not mean to. Lettuce, however, is not actually the best ketogenic food. It is low carb, but it is not high in fat so if you wanted to keep carbs low and eat it that would be fine, but it will not help you reach the fat goal you are wanting.

Food waste is also a really big problem that takes a toll on the environment. Fruits and vegetables tend to be one of the highest wasted foods at forty percent to the only thirty-three percent that meat does. That's only a seven percent difference but it does add up. Imagine for a moment that you have a family of four people. You are thinking you want to eat healthily, so you take your family to the grocery store and pick up healthy fruits and vegetables along with other items thinking you are making really good choices.

Now think a week ahead. If you got those fruits and vegetables close to their expiration date (which commonly happens in grocery stores), then it might not have lasted in the fridge and could have gone bad. Or if you bought too much and could not finish it all that might get wasted too. In most cases, families buy it thinking they would use it and it sits in the refrigerator and goes bad then they need to throw it out. Now, we're not saying that does not happen with meat as well. I am quite sure it does. However, meat can be frozen—and therefore, it lasts much longer than something that sits in the fridge or on the counter. One issue that makes these findings difficult is that it also varies from country to country with what people throw away and waste. Some things are agreed upon though and it is what makes the science easier to comprehend.

The livestock industry is another thing that could help the planet instead of hurting it. Even though it is hated by many people, it also creates a livelihood or jobs and means of support, for over one billion of the world's poor families and employs over one point three billion people. Without the livestock industry, those families would be out of a job and could not support themselves or their loved ones.

The planet has many poor countries. Some so poor that they feed their children dirt before they go to school because it is all their community has, and they are unable to feed their schools a proper lunch and some families have to feed their children that same dirt for dinner. Some so poor that they are dying without proper water or the water that they are drinking is so contaminated it may not be safe to drink. Others still, may work all day for practically nothing because they have economic issues. In some of these poor countries, they need all the meat they can get because they may not be able to nourish their people with anything else because they have nothing else available. The same situation is present in countries where grazing is efficient because they do not have any land that is suitable for growing or sustaining crops. So they would not have that option either.

Another reason it might not be the best idea that we all stop eating meat the planet would be overpopulated with animals and then the emissions would grow higher because they are still producing manure. Only now, there would be many more animals because they are still giving birth to multiple animals and we are feeding and taking care of them all. Then when they grow up, they too are giving birth to multiple animals and the cycle would continue over and over again. The land and grain that we need for people would be used to keep the animals alive. So there would not be enough food for the people, and there would not be enough for the animals either. This causes both species to be hurt. Many would think this a heartless view and others would agree that we should value animals too. We are not saying in this book that we do not care for the animals on the earth. We are simply presenting facts. Only you can be the judge of how you feel and what path you will take.

Remember those countries that do not have soil that can produce good crops? As people will be eating less meat on a vegetarian ketogenic diet, they will need to eat more plants. In those lands that have soil that will not produce anything, the sheep and cattle and goats are actually helping make that inedible grass useful to people by turning it into edible milk and meat for the people of that land. In some countries that milk and meat is their only source of protein and fat to keep them nourished. Protein is a very important part of any diet and not having enough can cause problems for your health. If you take the option of using those animals away when they are the only things those people have, what do they have left, if they do not have crops? They would have no way to nourish themselves.

Also, the cropland mostly used for nuts, fruits, and vegetables—which is a big staple in the vegetarian diet and ketogenic diet—is what is called cultivated cropland. Grazing cropland is another type of cropland. This cropland is usually unsuitable for attempting to grow crops but is actually really good at feeding animals that we use for food such as cattle. The last type of cropland that we have is called perennial cropland. This is good for grain, and hay and other types of crops that are alive year round. What they do is harvest these crops multiple times before dying. The reason the vegan diet sticks out here is that it is the only diet that does not use all of the lands. It specifically does not use perennial cropland which would waste the chance to produce more food for the people of the planet because it can be used to feed the animals that produce milk, meat, and other things that could help impoverished countries that desperately need it.

Since vegetarians eat more plants and they've cut out meat, one of the dangers that can arrive is that you notice you're lacking in nutrients. Men and women need nutrients to stay healthy and strong and lack of these nutrients can leave you feeling sick and can cause damaging health issues. For example, lack of iron can cause anemia and for some people, pills or even liquid iron is not enough, and they are not able to stomach it and you could end up needing an iron drip if it gets low enough. This can be a scary process for people because it is being placed directly in your veins. Other important nutrients you need are protein, calcium, zinc and vitamin B12. As a side note, if a vegetarian consumes something with too many calories and too many saturated fats instead of unsaturated fats, that can cause you to not eat enough nutrients as well.

Osteoporosis is another health issue that can arise. Calcium is a very important nutrient that you should not ignore—yet, unfortunately, there are many in the vegetarian lifestyle that does just that. This can cause your bones to become weak and result in fractures and damage you might not be able to repair at all. Ways to keep your calcium up as a vegetarian are to eat items like kale and Chinese cabbage or spinach and broccoli. High potassium items with high magnesium can reduce blood acidity. You can find items like this in the fruits and vegetables you eat now you would just need to check. Lowering the blood acidity is helpful because you are lowering the chances of excreting calcium through your urine.

Regardless of what you eat on this particular diet, you might still need a supplement if you are not getting the things you need for your body. For example, studies have shown that most vegetarians do not get enough vitamin D and may need to take a supplement to correct that. Or a vitamin B12 supplement as B12 is only found in animal products. Since this includes dairy products most vegetarians are usually alright, but some are not as they could be trying to transition further into this lifestyle or into veganism. If that's the case, they will need to take supplements to help regulate the amount in their body.

One of the biggest debates about the ketogenic diet is whether going into ketosis is safe. Ketosis can actually be dangerous when your ketones build up. It can lead to high levels of dehydration and it is said that it can change the chemical balance of your blood. Another problem is if ketosis goes too far the body can go into ketoacidosis. This is what happens when ketones build up in your blood. When they build up in your blood it becomes acidic. This can cause your body to go into ketoacidosis which can cause you to fall into a coma or even die. People with diabetes are especially susceptible to ketoacidosis if they do not take enough insulin or if they are injured or sick. People can also fall into ketoacidosis when they have an overactive thyroid, or it could be caused by starvation.

It is very important to understand that if you are feeling tired or have flushed skin, throwing up, confusion, pain in your stomach, fruity smelling breath, feeling thirsty, or even urinating a lot—these are all signs of ketoacidosis, and you should call a doctor right away. Especially as when you have diabetes, the symptoms may start slowing with throwing up, but the process speeds up quickly in just a few hours. So when you are in ketosis, you need to make very sure you do not fall into ketoacidosis because it can lead to fatal sickness.

Lastly, another reason to be cautious is that in a ketogenic diet your insulin levels begin to go down. This causes your body to shed water and sodium. When the body does this is beginning to do what is called reduced bloat. It can also cause dehydration and lightheadedness or constipation and headaches. Low sodium is bad for the body because if your sodium and electrolyte levels are low you can have muscle weakness and changes in blood pressure. More scarily, your heartbeat can become irregular.

Dehydration is also a big issue with the ketogenic diet because in the first two weeks, you are losing water and electrolytes. This is a diet that in the first two weeks in the adjustment period you may experience diarrhea. When the body gets diarrhea, you are losing vital water from your body—especially if it is happening repeatedly. To keep yourself from getting dehydrated you might need to drink about two liters or more a day. You should start when you begin cutting the carbs in your diet because of being ketogenic.

Most ketogenic people also make what is called a fat bomb. This is a very popular trend in the Keto world, but it may not be the safest one. The 'fat bombs' are usually high in the fat of course, with a moderate amount of either artificial or natural sweetness. Keto dieters usually refer to fat bombs as a treat, snack, or dessert. Some use it before a workout. Some use it as a fat dense snack or a way to curb their sweet tooth. With the Keto diet you are trying to cut sugar and carbs. You're trying to eat cleaner. These fat bombs are usually ninety percent fat or even more. The fat from these bombs commonly comes from coconut milk or from dairy. While most use it as a snack or dessert some actually use it for a meal replacement. There is so much fat in these bombs that the calories for a single one can be anywhere from two hundred and fifty calories to five hundred calories. We know that Keto dieters strive for higher fat but depending on your calorie intake for the day you are using a big chunk of your calories for a small little goodie.

The goal of the Keto diet is to achieve ketosis. When you reach for snacks like you would with a fat bomb it could mean you are not in a state of ketosis any longer. Meaning that fat bombs are basically promoting snacking unnecessarily. Boiled eggs are a better way to respond to hunger. Your body needs to take its own time on this diet, and there is no quick fix. If you suddenly begin to consume large amounts of fat that are not going to make you adjust quicker.

The Keto diet's success is the result of hormones. One hormone in specific as a matter of fact. It called leptin. Leptin reacting to a lack of blood sugar in your body results in your body using stored fat for energy. The fat consumed for the energy would be used before the stored fat. This means that the benefits of fat bombs are diminished in terms of fat loss. This is because while you could be maintaining ketosis, you are fueling your ketones with the wrong thing. You're fueling them with fat bombs instead of an extra arm, stomach, or thigh fat.

Insulin and Leptin are opposing hormones in your body. One tells the body to stop storing fat, the other tells the body to store fat. Many people are concerned with insulin and insulin resistance. But a higher priority needs to be given to leptin. In the human body, any hormone that you overproduce decreases the bodies sensitivity to it. So in a body that has excess fat, the hormone leptin is being overused. This means that the impact of leptin resistance in the body is the body not knowing how or when to stop storing fat. So the fat could come from frying oil or coconut oil, but it would not matter.

The people that are encouraging fat bombs and swearing by them fail to realize or recognize that leptin resistance in the body, though improved when you are in ketosis, is still a really serious hormonal adaptation. This adaptation is not going to be reversed by consuming high amounts of fat.

One big problem that many people encounter unfortunately is bad advice. If you go on social media, there are so many people trying to tell you how to live your life and how you should go about it. Now to be fair most of these people think that they are helping. Some of them are and they have done their research to make sure that they are giving good advice and they've talked to doctors to make sure that the information they are giving people is good information. Others, however, can be causing damage to people and making them sick. For example, one social media user says she only eats a certain number of calories a day. If you do your homework, you'll realize those are eating disorder levels and not healthy. As many young women and men watch her channel, this person could be potentially harming thousands of young people and they could think that eating disorders are alright when they are not.

Others on social media say that you can eat over five thousand calories a day, most of which are certain types of sugar, not work out and you will lose weight and not have health problems. That is simply not true and that can be potentially life-threatening advice. Some people have diabetes and that much sugar can put them into ketoacidosis which can be fatal. The scary part about this is for diabetics it can become fatal in a matter of hours. That's a terrifying thought. Even normal people who do not have any issues can be severely damaged by this advice. You can gain weight which causes many health problems on its own, you cannot ingest that many calories and not work out and expect that you will not put on any pounds at all. You will because you're consuming so many calories a day. There are many other problems with this advice as well and people should not follow extreme diets because it is not safe and its misleading to give people advice without making sure that it's safe for the people who are listening to you.

Everyone can get on social media these days. We live in a digital world and children and teenagers younger and younger are taking advice from the net and not their parents. This is not a good thing. There is so much information on the internet that is not true and even more that's dangerous to impressionable young minds. People on the net or social media say that they can say what they want and should not have to worry about what they say but they should. They are considered role models to people around the world and with a society so crazed about diets we need to understand what's real information that is the right information and what is false and dangerous to our health.

Another thing that nutritionists say is that if you want to slim down a ketogenic diet is not the best way to do this. It's considered extreme, and nutritionists warn that it may not be healthy. Others say that it is not sustainable for people and they believe it is just not a good diet for you. Since this diet is also low in fiber it is been said that that can cause digestive issues with your body. These kinds of problems may take a while to heal. So this is not something that you want to have to deal with if you do not have to. They believe if you do a more balanced diet it will be better for your future diets and goals.

Chapter 4

How to Approach a Vegetarian Diet and Beginning to Remove Meat from Your Diet

One thing that I have heard so many people worry and stress about when beginning to adopt a vegetarian diet is that they will miss the meat or that they are worried about how to get the protein and iron. I've even had so many friends think that they could not do it because they would miss meat so much, and they were scared that they would not be able to keep it up over time. The one thing I recommend the most is that if you are really worried about cutting meat from your diet, go slow. Also, if it helps, there are so many yummy alternatives to meat, and you can find them at just about any supermarket, which should make the switch even easier. Another thing to remind people is that once you begin adjusting to this diet, you will probably begin to crave meat less and less. Many people have said that they have been vegetarian for most of their lives and do not miss meat at all. Others say that they feel bad for the meat eaters who are missing out on what vegetarians enjoy.

36

A good tip to start out does not go cold turkey. No pun intended. When you go cold turkey without adequate preparation, you tend to be more likely to go back to eating meat and your old diet. Then you feel guilty and it can be a bad cycle. Removing it slowly over time is the best way to go about this because you're familiarizing your body to the new food and letting go of the old. Over time you'll notice that you are craving meat less frequently, and the switch will become easier. A good example to go with is let's say you are trying to cut sweets out of your diet. So you remove anything with sugar in your house. Then you start to eat healthy for maybe a few hours or a day and you begin to get cravings. The problem with many people is they get so hungry because they do not have the proper research about what to eat, that they end up going on a binge or running out to the nearest place with cookies. Then you feel guilty and ashamed which only hurts you and your progress as well as your emotional being. If you slip up, remember you are human. It can happen to anyone, and there is no reason to feel guilty or ashamed. Slip-ups happen. The best thing we can do is to try again on the diet and try your best not to slip up. It is also important to note that slip-ups will probably happen in the first couple of days and if they do it is alright. The important thing is that you're trying to better yourself and that you're wanting to change. This is a good thing. Reminding yourself of that will help guide you because you will be able to understand that the effort you're putting forth is something to be proud of and one day you will not slip up at all.

You should also begin adding to your diet before taking things away. Familiarize yourself with how you prepare your new food, how it is stored, and the uses they have. With studying you will see that many of your items can be used as multipurpose items. Olive oil is great for your skin and hair just as one example of how it can be used in a different way. You should start adding more vegetarian staples but keep in mind that you are both a vegetarian and ketogenic people. Not just one or the other. This means that there are certain things that ketogenic eat that vegetarians do not such as fish or meat—or for vegetarians, most eat beans or potatoes and starchy foods, but ketogenic people usually avoid them because of the high carb content. So when adding things to your diet, keep in mind what you need to avoid and what will bring the most benefits to your new lifestyle.

A fun way to get yourself used to this new lifestyle is to experiment with different recipes that sound good to you. You'll either realize that you like it and want to eat it again or maybe share it with the people around you if you live with others. Or maybe instead you'll be able to tell that it is something you do not like and would not want to try again. Or maybe it is just something you did not like cooking. In that case, if you liked the dish but did not like the work it took to prepare it, which happens to many people, that might lead you to a new restaurant that has the foods you can eat, and you might like how they prepare it. Once you begin experimenting and getting comfortable making the meals, it will become easier to adopt a new diet and find new foods that you like.

Or you can alter the recipes you already have and use on a daily basis. If you eat meals with meat make them vegetarian and then make them ketogenic or Keto for short. You are still eating a meal that you already enjoy it is just a different version of it. This can help you with your transition because it is just adapting things you're already used to. An example would be chili. Chili does not have to include meat at all but if you really want it, try a meat substitute. Since beans are not good for ketogenic because most of them are high in carbs, be sure to go through those carefully looking into the carb content and find a better option for that part of the diet as well. You could come up with an amazing recipe no one ever thought of before or you might be willing to try recipes that you would not before this.

The grocery stores can help too. Many stores have entire sections devoted to vegetarian or vegan foods and they can be adapted into the ketogenic diet. Since vegetarianism and veganism are on the rise and on the move people and companies are paying attention and learning to add those foods that are needed to their shelves. Look around your local grocery store to see if they have a section that just has the options you can eat. You are going to be opened to a variety of new snacks and foods. You'll probably see snacks that you've never thought to try. When looking at these snacks though be sure that there healthy. Looks can be deceiving though. Many of the snacks that look healthy but when you check the label you see that it is basically the fastest way to get you to bloat and gain weight. There might even be snacks that you've never heard of before. Your ethnic aisles in the grocery store are good for this as well. If you really look around, you can find some great stuff that tastes amazing and learn about new flavor combinations. Another bonus is that since you are still able to consume animal products on a vegetarian diet, and you can consume cheese, many stores now have a section that's just for cheese and it ranges from basic cheeses to super fancy cheeses. You will be able to learn about different textures and flavors. Some can be really interesting. I've even seen cheese mixed with cranberries or cheeses mixed with spices. All of them have different stats though so be sure to ask questions and make sure that you can eat them with your diet. This diet is a really interesting way to learn about your likes and dislikes and you can find yourself shopping an entirely new way.

Another tip I recommend is going to stores of other cultures like Asian stores. From personal experience, I can honestly say that the Asian stores in my town have amazing vegetables and they are cheaper than my local grocery store. Another cool thing was they had vegetables that I do not normally see in my regular grocery store and some I had never heard of but wanted to try. For example, I hardly ever see fresh mangos in my grocery store, but they have boxes of them in my local Asian store. The same is true for some melons. I have been able to find super sweet and healthy melon pieces, big enough for a snack or side with a meal, for as cheap as a dollar or a few cents above that. It was an amazing way to open my eyes to new foods. It is also good for people to see that eating healthy does not have to be expensive. Some people have families of two or three and spend at least three hundred in a store but if you shop around and shop smart you could actually find that this diet is pretty sustainable, and you might end up saving money because it makes you think on what you are actually going to eat, and it could help eliminate food waste.

Another thing Asian stores are good for is tea. You may be surprised to learn this, but you can drink tea, just do not add milk. Milk is too high in carbs because of the lactose. Plain black tea or green tea is ok for a ketogenic diet, but you need to drink it plain because you're trying to stay away from too much sugar as well. Another tip for tea drinkers is that you really need to check the bottles on the tea at stores and gas stations. Most of it is heavily sweetened with either sugar or artificial sweeteners, and there are only a few brands that carry a safe version for dieters. Likewise, if you are in the southern states of the United States you need to tell them unsweetened tea or they will assume you want sweet, and it's extremely sugary (to the point where I've seen glasses have a little sugar at the bottom of the glass).

I can also get other really healthy drinks that taste amazing or sweet treats that do not break my calorie budget or the other diet goals I've set for myself. It was finding all the Asian stores in my town that inspired me to look for other stores of other cultures as well to see if anything in their stores met might diet needs. Like a Turkish supermarket that had amazing new foods for me to try and opened my eyes to amazing new flavors. Or a Mediterranean shop that had some of the tastiest snacks my husband had ever had, and they did not harm his diet either. Best of all, all the people in the stores were friendly and helpful. It can really open your eyes to a whole new world in your own backyard and you can learn so much about the foods that other cultures make and how you can make them as well.

Now that you are adding more vegetarian options to your diet, you can start phasing out the meat options and other things you will not be eating anymore. Start with the easiest leaving the hardest for last. An example of why this is a good idea is to imagine that you are training for a marathon. You need a special diet and have to build endurance. You start easy and build up to the hard stuff. This is how you want to do your phasing. If you only like sausage but love steak, sausage is going to be way easier to give up than steak because your taste does not favor it in the same magnitude, and your taste buds most likely do not have it very often. In cases like that you might not even notice that you gave something up because you were not used to having it—whereas if you slowly work at giving these things up by the time, you are at stake. It should be easier because you've already gotten rid of all the other food items so that you are prepared, and it should not be as hard because you've already been experiencing how to do it and because you will know the process.

Set reasonable goals. I recommend that you start small. Try being a vegetarian ketogenic for a day. Then a week, and from there, move up to ten days. At around ten days you'll probably begin to notice things about your body like you've lost a little weight, not big numbers but probably a couple of pounds, which is a good start. You'll also probably notice you have increased energy and feel like you can do more. The important thing though, is that you'll realize if this is something you want to do and if this is something that you are able to stick to.

If you can do it for ten days, you can start to add more days on. Around thirty days the odds are if you've made it this far, you would not want to go back. Plus, going slowly like this gives your taste buds a chance to adjust. For example, have you ever promised yourself that you'd give up soda? So you gave it up for a week, but then thought I can do it for another week and then another. You did not want it after that right? You did not crave it anymore because when you phase it out of your system it usually takes a little bit for the cravings to go away but once they do you adjust and then you might begin to crave healthy things because you've been making better choices in food and your diet.

Planning meals will also be a great help as well. It prepares you for what's ahead and makes you more aware of what you are putting in your body and what you should not be putting in it. Learning these new things will benefit you so much because it also helps you take care of yourself better. Most people these days practically live on fast food or eating at restaurants. By cooking for yourself, you are being nutritious and in the long run probably saving hundreds of dollars.

It also makes you think outside of the box. You can learn about other cultures and their cuisines and find out all the new foods accessible to you. Chinese, Thai, and Indian cultures all have great vegetarian options and with a little ingenuity, they can be adapted to become ketogenic as well. Planning your meals also makes sure that you are being held accountable. I've recommending prepping as well. If you already have the food ready, then you should not want to go out and get other food because you'd waste it right? You would not want to waste something you spent your time and money on. Besides, chances are it is going to be a much healthier option than something you were going to get somewhere else.

Have you ever been to a farmer's market? They are really so much fun and have so many options for fresh produce. If you live alone it is a fun way to get out for a day and explore, or if you have a spouse or children it can be a fun date or family fun day. There is so much to do and see and they have tons of booths. Sometimes the booths even have samples and will let you try the food first. I've had friends go to a local farmer's market and they did not know what type of grape the woman was selling. She was kind and helpful enough to explain what it was, how it was grown and even the health benefits that came with it. Then she gave each of them one to try. It turned out the grapes were delicious. But if they had not asked, chances are they would have passed it up. So that is another important thing to remember. Ask questions and do not be afraid. Plus, it is local, so you are helping small businesses as well as helping yourself. They are full of amazing items, and you can get a really good price for them. Most do not mind if you haggle, but some do—so on this one, I recommend treading lightly. In my experience, I have never had to because the prices were more than fair, and the people were super friendly. Another great thing about them is that you have access to vegetables you might not find somewhere else and you can meet new like-minded people who have the same goals or ideas that you do. You might even find that you make new friends. Or you can learn new tricks to preparing the food.

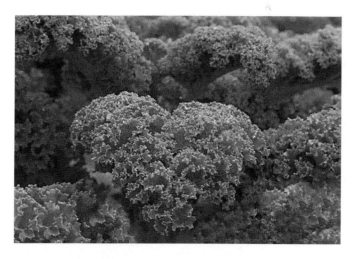

Have special food you can take with you when you leave your house. More and more places are trying to accommodate people's needs but some just do not have everything that you are able to eat because your diet can be a little bit restrictive. This is really going to help you keep yourself from being tempted by others influence or choices or if a place you are at cannot meet the needs of your diet. When you are out at social situations it can be tempted to get out of your diet or eat foods you know you should not. We have all been there. You can be at a dinner with a few friends and they want to share an appetizer and you think well one will not hurt, or they want to drink so you figure one drink will not have too many carbs or something along those lines, quick tip, a lot of drinks do have carbs and on a ketogenic diet it is really not recommended because you'll bust straight through your numbers. Some people even give in to the peer pressure because their friends get upset that someone is not eating like the rest of them. Ignore the peer pressure and do what you want to do. You do not have to answer to anyone but yourself. Having your own food or a plan will help you stay strong and stick to your diet in these cases.

Getting support will help you be able to stick to your diet as well. Having people around that love you and support you can be a very big help during this transition. Family can be a big help when you are making such a drastic change. If you are not able to be around encouraging people than be sure to find motivation and encourage yourself. Too many diets come with negativity and people making fun of people for trying something different. If this is what happens to you, I am sorry because no one deserves that at all and it can be very painful for someone to have to go through. The best thing you can do is ignore the hate and keep a positive attitude and remember what you are doing this for. You are doing this for you. Not them and you do not need their negativity. Ignore it and brush it off and stick to what you really want. I know it can be difficult but just remember you do not need to keep that negativity around you and you are stronger than they are. You are the one that lives your life, and you should be happy. Remember this and just keep pushing through. I recommend a reward for you as well. For instance, if you managed to stay a vegetarian ketogenic for a month reward yourself with something you've been wanting. Like a new pair of shoes or a movie that you've wanted to see. The act of giving yourself a reward will send a positive vibe to your brain that will reinforce your healthy habits and help you to want to keep going on your journey.

Chapter 5

Fundamental Nutrients and Micronutrients You Will Need as You Transition into the Vegetarian Ketogenic Diet

Nutrients and micronutrients are going to be really important for you in this lifestyle because missing out on them can make you really sick and cause deficiencies in your body that would need to be corrected right away because the deficiencies can cause some serious issues, and in some cases, life-threatening ones.

Micronutrients are nutrients that are needed for the human body. You usually need them in trace amounts. These micronutrients are part of development and growth. This is normal for the human body. This includes minerals, fatty acids, antioxidants, trace elements, and vitamins. Micronutrients in your body protect it from getting sick or help fight off diseases. They also ensure that the parts of your body under its care are being protected and functioning the way they are supposed to. This is a definite plus since they are in charge of almost every system in your body. A macronutrient, on the other hand, is a substance that is required in relatively large amounts by living organisms. Another way of describing it would be a type of food as a protein, fat, or carbs, which are required in large amounts in the human diet.

A perfect example is processed food. Take cookies for example. A popular brand contains virtually zero micronutrients. Instead, it is mainly composed of carbohydrates meaning it is something to steer clear of on a ketogenic diet. They can also drastically spike your blood sugar. On the other side of this spectrum, foods such as pastured eggs and leafy greens that you can consume on this diet are a great way to get your micronutrients. They include vitamin A, omega threes, and potassium.

The reason that making sure you are getting your essential vitamins is that on the ketogenic diet, can be low in micros if you are only trying to hit certain goals and not all of them. One thing to remember is that you need both your micronutrients and macronutrients. You still need micronutrients and their value in your diet. Knowing how to compose meals that are rich in nutrients is important and will be a key factor in this diet and vegetables are really going to help you get them in, as they are full of them.

Your body is transitioning in this diet as well. If you are not watching your intake you may end up deficient in one or many things and this will harm your health. You can even go through what is called the Keto flu.

The Keto flu is what happens when your body begins adjusting to running on a different ratio of macronutrients than it used to. You begin to experience flu-like symptoms and experience stomach pain, dizziness, brain fog, diarrhea, constipation, muscle cramps, trouble sleeping, sugar cravings, the inability to stay asleep, or lack of focus and concentration. This does not happen to everyone, but it is something to be aware of.

Vegetarians need calcium and vitamin D especially. Calcium is vital for maintaining strong bones and teeth. As you are still eating and consuming dairy foods on this diet you will be able to get calcium into your system pretty easily. Greens are also a good source of calcium. Broccoli and kale are really good examples. Another is turnips and collard greens. Just remember what veggies are best for the ketogenic diet as well. In a ketogenic diet in the early stages when you are losing more calcium because of the transitioning process where you are losing electrolytes, you will need more amounts of calcium, as you are losing that too.

Vitamin D is also good for bone health. Since milk is high in both sugar and carbs and not good for ketogenic you should try to find your vitamin D in cereal if you can. If you are still not getting enough vitamin D and if you do not get out in the sun much, you will probably need a supplement to help you get the right amount. They offer plant derived ones as well if you are trying to remove more animal products from your diet.

Vitamin B12 or cyanocobalamin is necessary to produce red blood cells. This vitamin is important because it forms the red blood cells in your body. It also helps with the fatty acids in your body by breaking them down to produce vital energy that you will be able to use throughout your day. It is the most well-known B vitamin for a reason. It is also helpful with mental clarity and used to prevent anemia. Anemia is a condition that happens when you have a red blood cell deficiency. Or a deficiency of hemoglobin in the blood. This results in weariness and pallor. Pallor means you have an unhealthy pale appearance. So vitamin D is going to be a big issue if you are not getting enough as anemia can cause an entire host of problems. On a vegetarian ketogenic diet, you get some leeway here. Eggs and milk both contain b12. It is not generally found in plant foods, but you can find it in fortified breakfast cereals. You can also find it in some yogurts, which is also a good food to consume. If you find that you are not getting the amount that you need with these foods, you will need to find a supplement to correct it.

Zinc is important for your body because it has a part in the formations of the proteins in your body as well as playing a role in cell division. It also has a part to play as an elemental part of the enzymes that are inside you. Zinc is more easily absorbed from animal products, but it can be absorbed from plant sources as well. Just not quite as easily. Cheese is a really good option for zinc for an animal product option. For a plant source of zinc, you've got choices from whole grains, wheat germ, soy products, and nuts. Most nuts are high in carbs though, so you might not want to choose that option unless you are willing to possibly go to high in carbohydrates.

Iron is crucial as a component of red blood cells. For ketogenic people, your options are a little more limited on this because beans, peas, and lentils are all high in carbohydrates and should be avoided or if you absolutely love them, in very sparing amounts. Whole grain products are a good source of iron, but the same adage is true here as well. Some, not all, whole grain options have a high percentage of carbs, so you really need to read your labels and know what you are buying before you eat it. Dark leafy green vegetables are a good option that you can eat, however. Many of the greens that have been mentioned in previous chapters can be a good source of iron as well as having other benefits. Something that you'll have to remember though is iron does not absorb easily from sources that come from plants very well. Iron absorbs much more easily from animal sources and for this reason, it is recommended that vegetarians need more iron than non-vegetarians and that they should try and make sure to up their intake. A way to help your body absorb iron you should eat foods that are high in iron and other vitamins like vitamin C especially. When people do not have enough iron in their bodies, they can develop anemia—and if your iron gets too low, you may need a blood transfusion.

Omega three fatty acids have an integral part in your new diet and health as well. Omega threes are important for the health of your heart. They are also helpful with brain development, making sure that the oxygen your body needs is getting into the bloodstream, reducing inflammation and helping your blood pressure be stable or lowering it if necessary. Omega threes are mostly in fish and eggs. While you cannot consume fish, you can consume eggs. Diets that do not include these items are usually not as high in omega three's as they need to be and the active form of this may be low. For vegetarian ketogenic, there are a couple issues with how to get them in your system. As long as you monitor your soy intake carefully studies say you should be alright as there are still debates about whether it can cause cancer and other effects if you are trying to get your omega three's using soy. Some studies show that there are no adverse effects so more research is needed to be conclusive. You can get it in ground flaxseed, which is also a good source.

Iodine is a vital mineral because it is going to help you with your thyroid gland. Iodine helps regulate thyroid hormone levels and could help with the condition known as hypothyroidism. This is a serious condition that can cause some pretty big problems in your health. It can cause superficial problems to your skin, or it could cause more serious health issues like making you pack on the pounds or experience weakness in your body. They add iodine to processed table salt so it is pretty easy to come by. Seaweed has iodine as well and is rich in vitamins and minerals that can help support the immune system and balance hormones. Dulles is another sea vegetable that contains iodine and is rich in vitamins and minerals. In many of the cases of vegetarianism and ketogenic diets, a supplement can help correct any deficiencies you might have.

Vitamin K is another crucial vitamin. It makes sure your bones get the calcium they need. It is an important part of the coagulation of your blood and it works as a transporter as well by getting calcium for your bones from your bloodstream. Examples of this are kale, Brussel sprouts, broccoli, and spinach. Eggs are also a good source of vitamin K. If you eat enough of these items, you should not be lacking with this vitamin.

Phosphorus does a lot for your body. Your body has hundreds of cells. Each of those cells has a function and phosphorus is involved in hundreds of them like a mom who's always trying to get in your business, phosphorus is in your functions. These work to help you improve digestion, boost energy levels, make sure that you are able to utilize nutrients better, and help in the process of balancing hormones in your body. By making sure you are getting the right amount into your system you can make sure your level of phosphorus does not go to low as this can cause problems like weak bones, tooth decay. Trouble concentrating and anxiety. Two good examples of phosphorus are broccoli and eggs.

Vitamin C prevents bad cholesterol from causing untold damage to your system. Another function it performs is that it works as an antioxidant. Vitamin C is an important part of your body's dealings with collagen. It helps you use it and make sure you have more of it. This is a good thing because it helps your muscles, which are obviously an important part of your body and it helps strengthen your blood. A lot of low-carb options have vitamin C. Spinach, broccoli, kale, and cauliflower all have vitamin C. Brussel sprouts are a good source of vitamin C as well. This debunks a lot of the ideas of where the best place to get vitamin C, but these are the options that are best for a ketogenic.

Magnesium is responsible for so much in our bodies. Believe it or not, our bodies have biochemical functions. This is where magnesium comes in. Magnesium is responsible for them. But the number is what might surprise you. It is responsible for a vast amount of the ones we have. Over three hundred in fact. So if you are not getting enough, imagine the damage it could do. This is an electrolyte and a mineral, and it is also a vital part of the process known as the synthesis of protein. It is involved in the production of many things in the body like cell reproduction, energy and how certain things form. Like fatty acids. Muscle cramping is the most common of the symptoms of lacking in magnesium. Other things you could experience are fatigue and dizziness. Cooked spinach is high in magnesium at around one hundred and sixty milligrams. When you are tracking your magnesium and making sure you hit the right number, you'll see what type of foods the best for this are and how much you'll need to consume.

Sodium is one of the biggest electrolytes that you as a ketogenic starting this diet can become deficient in. Since it is also a mineral it is an important thing to be aware of. There is a debate on how much sodium we need, and some people choose to avoid sodium at all costs. Others believe this is a nutrition fallacy. In previous studies, it was thought to exacerbate cardiovascular disease. There are many new studies now that are disproving this idea. Sodium is important because it helps retains normal levels of water in our bodies and controlling blood pressure. It also helps our bodies absorb micronutrients.

The ketogenic diet is eliminating a large number of carbs in your body. This means it has a diuretic effect. In case you are unaware, a diuretic is classified as any substance that promotes what is called diuresis. Diuresis is the increased production of urine. So when you are in ketosis or beginning to enter it, you are shedding what you need in your body, and you will have to find a way to get that water back. You will also need those electrolytes back because of they are so vital to your system. If you are an athlete on this diet, due to the strenuous activities you perform regularly you will lose even more sodium because of your sweating. So your sodium is escaping through your sweat. If you are obese or overweight, you are probably storing too much sodium from your insulin levels. Obese and overweight people can have chronically high levels of insulin. So a sedentary lifestyle would not need to consume as much sodium as an athlete. If you have low sodium, you can be unable to perform a strenuous activity and suffer from headaches or extreme fatigue.

When you begin the ketogenic diet the first couple of weeks are where you really need to monitor your sodium. While your body is transitioning during this time it really is losing what it needs so be sure to keep an eye on it. Most people on diets exercise as well and if you are you will need to watch even closer.

Potassium is another thing you might lose on this diet. When you are losing the sodium in your system you begin to lose potassium. Potassium-deficient people can have a loss in muscle mass, skin problems, physical weakness, constipation, and irritability. If your defiance gets to be too bad it can cause problems to the heart. Such as irregular heartbeat or it can have potentially life threating issues like heart failure. Mushrooms, spinach, avocados, and kale are all good sources of potassium. One cup of spinach has about eight hundred and forty milligrams, one cup of kale has five hundred milligrams of potassium, one cup of mushrooms has four hundred and twenty milligrams while one avocado has one thousand milligrams.

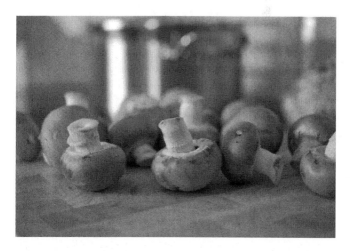

Vitamin A is going to be vital for several functions in your body. Some of the functions it performs are organ growth, proper vision, and cell reproduction. Since you are in a ketogenic diet you should be getting plenty of vitamin A. You can get it in kale, broccoli, spinach, eggs, and dairy products. On this one, studies have been showing that supplementing is probably not wise here is that the ketogenic diet restricts carbs. When you restrict carbs to this level the need in the body for vitamin A is also decreased.

Continuing down the list B vitamins are next. You can use supplement available just about anywhere to get all of the types of B vitamins is one pill. This might help you because there are seven main types. The ketogenic diet consumes large leafy green vegetables, which is good. But in most cases, they are also consuming meat. In this diet, we are not so we may actually fall into the case of needing a little help. If you remember to consume a lot of green leafy vegetables and a large volume of them, studies show you may still be alright. This is why it is important to keep monitoring your intake and knowing how much you need.

The most essential and common B vitamins are:

Vitamin B1 which is called Thiamin. Thiamin is essential in creating energy or the ATP. It is necessary for nerve cell functioning and it is crucial to the breakdown of proteins, fats, and carbs. A lot of good ketogenic options that contain vitamin B1, unfortunately, are meat options. But one option that is ok for you as a ketogenic and vegetarian is nuts.

Vitamin B2 or Riboflavin. Riboflavin can sometimes work as an antioxidant and helps convert macronutrients in your body to energy. It helps in processing amino acids and fats as well. Cheese is a good option here because there are so many different kinds. Cheddar cheese and feta cheese are good for vitamin B2. Raw or cooked mushrooms are a good option as well as cooked spinach and eggs.

Vitamin B3 is called Niacin. B3 helps with memory function and supports healthy skin central nervous system functioning and helps improve sex hormones. Another thing its useful for is your body has what's called cell reparation. What it does is release the energy from the macros in your body. Niacin is helping to release that energy for you to rely on. Like vitamin B1, most of the good ketogenic options for optimal nutrient absorption is from meat. Do not despair though. There are still options for vegetarians and they include mushrooms which can contain about two point five milligrams of niacin per cup, cheddar cheese, and cooked eggs. Another good option is avocados. One medium avocado can contain about three point five milligrams of niacin.

Vitamin B5 is known as pantothenic acid. This acid is an integral vitamin that will help with your fats by extracting the energy from them. They also help produce steroid hormones and red blood cells. Avocados have healthy fats and are a good source of this particular vitamin. Shitake mushrooms might be another good choice. They do have about four point five net carbs per one hundred grams, so you might have to limit how many you eat depending on what your intake of carbs is. Eggs are another good option

59

and if you opt for free-range eggs you will be able to consume even more nutrients like beta-carotene and omega threes but less cholesterol. Portobello mushrooms are debated to have about two point two grams of carbs, so you might have to watch those as well.

Vitamin B6 is pyridoxine and influences your brain processes. Like other vitamins that help with your red blood cell formations, this one does too. It also helps with the metabolism of your carbohydrates and protein. However too much in your body can be toxic. Now overdosing on B6 with natural food is rare but it is possible if you are on a supplement. If you have too much in your body, you can have muscle spasms and cramps, experience permanent nerve damage which of course can impact your mobility. It can also cause irritation to the nerves in your brain and around your brain which can cause migraines and headaches. Fatigue is common as well because the toxicity can cause disruption to your sleep cycles and cause insomnia. You can also experience depression, irritability, stress, and anxiety. Making sure you have the right amount is crucial. Avocados are useful here as well as they contain point four milligrams of vitamin B6.

Vitamin B7 is known as biotin. Biotin contributes to regulating your blood cholesterol levels. It is vital to your energy metabolism. It is also critical for fat synthesis and a necessary part of amino acid metabolism. There has also been some evidence to show that vitamin B7 may be able to reduce triglyceride levels in your blood. This will help lower cholesterol levels and may improve heart function. There are possible side effects here as well. If you take too much in a supplement you can experience issues with your thyroid. You can also experience digestive issues. It can also interact with other medications such as anti-seizure medications. Eggs and nuts are helpful in getting B7 in your system. You've also got the options of spinach some evidence says you should try boiled, fresh, broccoli and mushrooms. Cheddar cheese has about point four micrograms. Milk would be another source, but it is not allowed on a Keto diet because of carbs and sugar so you'll need to stick with other options.

Vitamin B9 is folate. Folate is needed for women who are with child. Folate helps the development of the fetal cell growth and nervous system and women who are carrying a child should consumer larger amounts of folate for that reason. Pregnant women need to especially make sure that they are consuming enough not just for them but for their unborn children. Another reason folate is important is that it also helps those formations again for the red blood cells. The function of red blood cells is to get oxygen around your body to all the places it needs to be. Red blood cells carry them there. Good sources of folate are Brussel sprouts. Others include broccoli and spinach.

The last important B vitamin is B12, which is mentioned above. It is important to get enough in the B vitamins because deficiencies in them may cause psychological disorders like paranoia, anger, confusion, anxiety, and depression. It has been linked to difficulty walking, insomnia, tingling can appear in body parts and palpitations of your heart may begin to occur as well.

Foods that are high in a variety of the B vitamins on this list are nuts, leafy green vegetables, and dairy products.

Chloride is a big component of salt, so you are most likely not lacking this in a ketogenic diet. But you may need a little more when you first start out because your body is going to be flushing out electrolytes.

Chromium is a little tricky. It is not found in large quantities and it is also not found in large quantities in very many foods that you eat. The most abundant food that it appears it is broccoli and even then, half a cup only contains eleven micrograms per serving. This is only about one-third of your daily needs, but it is the one that contains the most. Reports of a chromium deficiency are rare because it is scarce in a ketogenic diet it is possible that one might occur.

Copper is one of the nutrients you should not really have to worry about on a ketogenic diet because of all of the green vegetables you will be eating. It is pretty abundant in a ketogenic diet because it also shows up in nuts.

Fluoride is present and actually most abundant in water. There is also a high content in dairy, greens, and avocados so this is another thing you should not have to worry about in your diet because you'll be getting what you need.

Manganese is similar to magnesium and shows up in nuts that you will be able to eat, and evidence shows that this is something your diet should not be lacking either but it is still important to know about.

Sulfur mostly comes from animal products. Eggs are a good way to get some in your system and most of the sulfur-containing veggies are totally okay on a ketogenic diet, so this is something that you should not be lacking either.

Fiber is something that you should try to get from food. Not supplements. Fiber is useful, but some believe it may not be as healthy as we've been told. Fiber is not found in any animal products but rather it is a plant consumption indicator. Fiber is fermented into fat by the bacteria in a human gut. Staple foods in a ketogenic diet such as nuts and avocados are quite high in fiber. If you add in some green vegetables and you should be even better. To make sure you get the last bit, then you need to try eating something like flaxseeds, and low carb flours. That should boost you to the amount you need. Watch your intake, and you should not lack in fiber on either a vegetarian or ketogenic diet if you make sure to do it right.

Selenium is also something to watch while you are on this diet, but you do not need to think about this one too hard. Selenium is essential for fertility and your thyroid gland. But guess what this is such an interesting way you can get your selenium and its super easy. Since we only need a little bit of selenium for our diets, one single brazil nut has one hundred percent of your daily need. Simple right?

Molybdenum is another easy one that you do not really need to worry about. Most people get enough without even trying. It has actually been shown if you have too much it can increase your copper excretion. Nuts are the best source of molybdenum on the ketogenic diet and the only way you would have to worry is if you do not consume them at all. You just need to remember which nuts are low in carbs and which are high in carbs.

Now in the description of the nutrients above, I have mentioned if you are not getting enough of them you might need a supplement to help you get the right amount. An important thing to remember on this though is that supplements are not designed to replace food. Micronutrients from natural whole foods are the best idea for getting your nutrients instead of relying on supplements.

Supplements also do not contain the carotenoids, antioxidants or flavonoids that come with eating natural food. The nutrients you need for your body are not as potent with a supplement as they are with food. They become the most potent when you get them from the food you eat. You should aim to get your macros from good whole food. This will keep you on the right track. By consuming whole foods, you are also consuming a larger variety of protective substances such as antioxidants. It also helps you consume fiber. Supplements may also cause excess micronutrients that are excreted through your urine versus absorbing the nutrients more effectively with the whole foods.

Food quality matters here as well. Regular food has hormones, but organic does not have any hormones and go through a rigorous process to make sure that the organic food you buy is of high quality. It also usually has more macros that you need, and the density of the nutrients is higher. Organic food is also raised and grown with fewer pesticides, which is the reason that they are usually more expensive. A good example is a study from about four years ago. It was discovered that certain organic crops have more antioxidants than produce that was not organic. Now a few of those things you cannot eat, but the rest we can on this diet and it is nice to know that the organic version is better for our body.

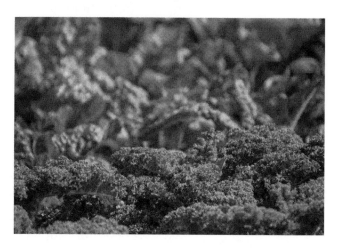

Now while you should concentrate on getting your nutrients from food, which is good because this is the greatest way to make sure you are running at your bet and have the proper amounts in your body. While it is not recommended to rely on supplements alone you can still use them if you need them. While having any of the issues, I am about to list than you might want to consider taking a supplement.

If you are aged fifty and up. Older than fifty will usually need to do this.

You need to consume a variety of different foods. A wide amount. If you do not or are restricting your calories too much, you will need to do this to help regulate your system by getting it where it should be.

If you are pregnant and are unable to sustain a complete micronutrient profile because you cannot eat enough. It is also important to mention that pregnant women need to be more mindful of the nutrients in their body both macro and micro because if you are pregnant, it is not just you—you need to watch out, for it is your unborn child as well, and they need the vitamins you are going to be providing him or her. You'll need to monitor your intake to make sure you are getting what you need.

If you are not in the sun enough. A supplement will be important here if you do not go out and get some sun on you or get it from food.

If your body is not absorbing nutrients properly

because you are sick with a condition that does not let your body absorb the nutrients the manners the body is supposed to.

Those following a vegetarian diet or lifestyle.

If you follow the vegetarian ketogenic diet the right way and follow it correctly, it can provide your body with everything you need. You need to track your intake very carefully to make sure that you do not have prolonged symptoms of the Keto flu because in the first few weeks it is likely that you will experience at least a few of the symptoms as your body is adjusting. If you follow it incorrectly you could end up hurting yourself and your health.

Another tip is to remember not to get your calories from foods that have no micronutrient value or too little value. Fill up instead of organic and healthy foods because they have more benefits for your body and dietary needs. A multivitamin can also fill in any gaps in nutrition. If all else fails, consult your doctor. There have been some doctors that have said if you still have symptoms like aches and weakness for longer than two weeks you should even consider ending the diet completely, but your doctor will be able to tell what is best for you.

Chapter 6

The Best Sources of Fat and Protein

Now, since you are adopting the vegetarian lifestyle, you obviously will not be getting your protein from meat. This means that you are going to have to get it from somewhere else. Protein is very important in any diet—meatless or not—and if you do not have enough, you can experience many health issues that I am sure you would rather avoid. Many people are confused on how much protein we actually need—and while research studies and articles often disagree on the subject, there are those that believe that we do not need as much as we have been told. Make sure that you know the proper amount that you need before adopting this diet. This lifestyle is really going to take research because the vegetarian diet and ketogenic diet have so much involved. With this book, we've taken out the guesswork—but you are still going to need to figure out how much of things like protein and vitamin A and things of that nature because everyone is different, and people who exercise more like athletes who live an active lifestyle are going to be different than people who live a sedentary lifestyle.

Since you are adding the ketogenic diet to your vegetarian one some of the protein sources that a vegetarian would be able to use you will not be able to because they are high in carbs and so they would not be able to help you on this diet as it goes against the percentages from the ketogenic side. There are some beans that would be a great staple for a vegetarian but not a ketogenic because the amount of carbs maxes you out for the day. Some examples of this are peas, lentils, and chickpeas. These are usually great options for a meatless diet because they are so versatile, but for the carbs on a ketogenic diet, they are red flagged as something you should not eat. Chickpeas yield about thirty-two point five grams in net carbs, which for almost any ketogenic diet would be your whole days take in just one sitting and then you have nothing left for the rest of the day because you already maxed yourself out. Peas are another no-go because they have seventeen points two, which is also way too high. While lentils taste great, they are going to be something you need to pass up as well because they have twenty-eight grams in net carbs. To add insult to injury these are all great sources of protein which were going to need in this diet. But no worries. We found a lot of protein options that are low carb and perfect for your new diet. Thankfully, there is a lot we can still choose from. One thing to remember as well is that it is recommended that since you are trying to put your body into ketosis for this diet you should not eat too much protein because it can interfere with that though you still need to make sure you get the right amount into your system. It has been recommended by some doctors that you should get no more than twenty percent of your daily calories from protein sources that are plant-based.

Missing meat or having a craving you cannot ignore? Try this on for size. Vegan 'meats' are a great substitute for real meat in a vegetarian or vegan diet. Some of the most popular are tofu, tempeh, and seitan. These are wonderful for protein and great for ketogenic people because the carb factor is super low. On the other side of this though, a lot of the other fake meats are super high in fat, which is not a problem, but they are also high in carbs. You'll need to learn how to identify ingredients and make sure you are not wasting money on something that you will not be able to eat. To clarify tofu is made of soy milk that has been condensed and pressed into a white block. Kind of the same process they use to make cheese. Now while soy is healthy for you, nutritionists and doctors have said that you need to watch how much you are eating because recent studies have shown that soy may cause certain types of cancer. Tofu and tempeh, which is the next fake meat were going to mention, both contain soy, and there are more than just possible cancer-causing elements. Soy also contains what are called goitrogens. A goitrogen is a plant compound that can impair how your thyroid functions. If you experience cold sensitivity, constipation, or dry skin, fatigue or weight gain as a result of upping your soy-based products you should begin to limit the amount of soy you are eating. Another great thing about tofu is it has the ability to absorb the flavor from sauces. This is really beneficial because there are so many recipes that contain meat that will not be available to you but now you can try them and switch out the meat for tofu.

Tempeh is considered an Indonesian food staple. The process of making tempeh is fermenting soybeans in banana leaves. You need to leave them in until firm earthy patty forms. It has been considered a meat substitute since the twelfth century and uses in a multitude of dishes. It is also a great source of protein. They say one cup of tempeh is about thirty-one grams of protein. Another bonus? Its taste is a mild nutty flavor that can work amazingly well in many different recipes and cultures.

Seitan is usually referred to as wheat gluten. It began to appear in the sixth century. It was used as an ingredient in Asian cuisine. It has been a good substitute for meat for over a thousand years. Traditionally it was the product of people rinsing and cooking the wheat dough. This removed the starch and instead left a protein dense substance that people quickly realized made an amazing meat substitute. If you like knowing nutritional facts, you love this one. Its cholesterol-free, low carb, perfect for ketogenic people, and the protein is sixty grams per cup! On this one, you really cannot go wrong—it has everything you need.

It is very likely that you will not just be eating fake meat for every meal so you are also going to need to get some protein veggies and other sources of protein too. Eggs are packed with protein and healthy fats making it a great food for the ketogenic diet because it is so high fat low carb and it can be used in just about anything. You can use eggs for wraps, sandwiches, tostadas, you can use them on salads or even just have hardboiled eggs for a snack. Cheese is a great product that is both high in fat but a good source of protein. Plus, its low in carbs making it a perfect choice because it will be a great addition to your diet because it plays to those percentages. This is another one that you can use in literally almost anything. If you combine the hardboiled eggs with some cheese and vegetables, you have a small meal or an awesome snack. Most vegetarians and vegans think that nuts are a big source of the diet and while they do not have to be its honestly a good idea for a vegetarian ketogenic diet because nuts like walnuts have about six grams of protein and only two point eight in carbs. Yogurt is a good option as well. If really like yogurt though, check out Greek yogurt as opposed to regular yogurt. Greek yogurt has got more protein than regular yogurt and since it is got the healthy fats you need it keeps you fuller longer. This is a good thing because if you are not hungry then chances are you not bingeing or worse bingeing on unhealthy foods.

Now for some of the vegetables that can help with your diet. Greens are chocked full of protein and they can really help boost your diet and your system. Spinach is a great source of protein at two point nine grams per one hundred grams of protein, and it is a great alternative to lettuce for salads or even sandwiches. It has a really good taste as well and it is a versatile ingredient that can also be used in breakfast recipes as well. Brussel sprouts are another good source at three-point-four per hundred grams of protein and since many people say it is an acquired taste the internet has gone crazy coming up with good recipes to make the taste better—and now, there are a ton of people worldwide that cannot get enough making them a new popular food. Kale is another super green. It is being put in everything from juices for cleansing and detoxing, salads, muffins, which most people would not think about, all kinds of new things, and it contains a whopping four point three grams of protein which tops the list that was going through.

One of my personal favorite foods is mushrooms. Now, they get a bad rap because people have preconceived notions about mushrooms which I understand. But make up your own mind, and you'll see they taste amazing. These are good for your diet as well as three-point-one grams of protein and they can be used in just about anything. You can use them for snacks, salads, stir fry's, you can use them on sandwiches or a great option is to go for a veggie burger with mushrooms. Not only that—there is a variety of mushrooms that will be good on this diet, and they all can make a recipe so much better.

Zucchini is also a good option that helps with other vitamin and nutrients that you need on this diet as well as cauliflower and avocado. One thing these all have in common is it is also a great source of vitamin

C. Zucchini has come up so fast in many diets these days, and there are so many cool ways you can cook it and use it in your diet. Do you like spaghetti? It is something you would have had to give up but now you do not! You can actually turn zucchini into noodles. It is actually really easy and is a great alternative to pasta because it fits perfectly with your new diet. This is how you start taking old recipes and changing them for new ideas.

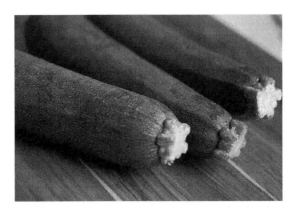

Another thing that you need in this diet is fat. The percentage ratio for this diet is very high so you'll need a good variety of foods to get to the number you need. A good source of fat is cooking oil. A lot of people with special diets end up cooking for themselves. That's going to help you here as most cooking oils are high in the healthy fats you need. If you want to bake or fry things it recommended you use avocado oil since it has a very high smoke point. Coconut oil is a great source if you need a 'fat bomb' like desserts or if you are looking for a recipe that bakes under three hundred and fifty degrees. One of the healthiest oils you can use is olive oil. A warning though, at four hundred and five degrees Fahrenheit the oil becomes less healthy because it oxidizes. Olive oil has no carbs because it is a pure source of fat. It is a great base for a healthy mayonnaise or salad dressing.

Red palm oil is a popular choice as well because it is a great way to get vitamin A and E because its rich in it. It has a buttery-like texture and a mild carrot flavor, but let it be a warning that needs to be said about this oil is that palm oil's making process is done in such a way that it causes devastating effects. When they make palm oil many of them are made in a way that devastates wildlife and their environment. It is recommended that if you really need or want this oil in your diet, make sure you buy oil that is from the certified sustainable palm oil products. Or RSPO certified products because these are a better option.

Many of the foods you eat are going to have great fat numbers as well. Avocados, nuts, and seeds are all good in healthy fats, but you still need to watch out. Cashews are high in carbs and you want to stay low, so this is either something or going to have to cut out or make sure you eat less of them. Seeds are also higher in inflammatory omega six fats. It is not recommended to lean on them or rely on them for a dietary fat staple.

You can also use coconut cream and milk for high-fat content and delicious flavor for many recipes and dishes. Butter has long been told to everyone that it is an enemy because it is so high in fat. In this diet, you can use it if you'd like because you are trying to get to that high-fat content percentage. Like in any situation you should use the butter in moderation, but it is still nice to be able to use it in your diet and the recipes you are going to want to be able to use.

Cheese is also good for fat—the healthy fat, of course, and there are hundreds of different kinds. They are very low in carbs but high in fat. This is perfect for your needs. You can use cheese in so many different ways that it is the perfect staple. You can use it at all three meals and use it for snacks. How can you go wrong? Some of the most common cheeses that you can use are cheddar, brie, goat cheese or cream cheese. Or mozzarella. You can have so much fun coming up with unique ways to use these cheeses in your diet.

Nut butter also plays to those percentages on the high-fat side, especially if you are trying to steer away from animal products. Nut butter is a delicious option for vegetarians, and it can go on anything. I've even seen people use it on pizza before, to name one interesting combination. They are great for snacks, smoothies, Asian cuisine, and many other interesting food dishes. This is something that should be in every vegetarian ketogenic diet because it is so versatile.

Dairy items have fat in them too which makes them a helpful choice. Some of the most popular that people use are yogurt or cream. Just as there are hundreds of different options for cheese, there are at least a couple of dozen different types of yogurt. You can get yogurt simply for the fat or go for a combo and use the yogurt for protein and fat. Cream can also be very versatile. Most people think cream is for things like breakfast foods or deserts, but there are so many recipes that include cream and are savory and rich or that can fill you up so well you are not hungry for hours. Cottage cheese is a good source of fat that tastes good as well. It can be served with eggs, vegetables and makes a really good snack to keep you full in between meals.

Olives are a good source of nondairy fat. Like the other items on this list it may be considered a side food or item, but it can be added to literally anything, though most of them do use it as a complimentary item or an appetizer instead of using it with full meals. It contains the antioxidant oleuropein which may protect your cells from damage because it has anti-inflammatory properties. Studies also suggest that eating olives may help decrease blood pressure and may prevent one loss. A one-ounce serving contains two grams of carbs. The math for this works to one gram of carbs for about seven to ten olives.

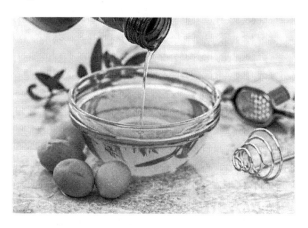

Chapter 7

Vegetarian Ketogenic Diet Recipes and Meal Plans

Breakfast

Now that you have all this information about how to eat a vegetarian ketogenic diet, you need some good recipes to help you realize all the good food you can eat and some meal plans to make it even easier on you.

Breakfast is our first meal—and depending on how you do it, you can be energized for the rest of the day or crash because you have not eaten a proper meal. I wanted to find a really good breakfast bowl because I like breakfast bowls and because know that there are a lot of people out there who love them as well. Breakfast bowls are a great thing to do for mornings because they are simple and because you can pack them full of the vitamins you need to get your day started on the right foot.

This breakfast bowl has gotten a variety of vegetables, and you get to enjoy a little salsa with it, which is great for a spicy kick. I love adding salsa to any meal because there are some great low-calorie options out there that do not weigh down the meal with unnecessary things that we do not need, but we get an explosion of flavor that just adds a nice *feel* to a meal. Salsa is also well-known for being made of vegetables, and that is good for your diet, as many of them contain the nutrients you'll need.

Very-Veggie Cauliflower Hash Brown Breakfast Bowl

free gluten low lowvegetarian20 minute meal
Servings: 1

Ingredients:

- 1.5 avocado
- 1.5 lime
- 1 small handful baby spinach
- pepper
- 2 eggs
- salsa
- garlic powder
- 1 or one and a half cups cauliflower rice
- mushrooms – sliced four ounces
- extra virgin olive oil
- 1 green onion, chopped

Instructions:

1. Adding in pepper and salt to the bowl, mix them with the two eggs. This mixture will be used in a short while.

2. Whisk eggs with salt and pepper in a small bowl then set aside for a little bit later.

3. Add avocado, the pepper, lemon or lime juice, and garlic powder and continue the process until you come up with a mashed mixture. This will be used in a short while.

4. Through medium setting, in a ten-inch skillet, cook a sprinkle of additional virgin olive oil together with four ounces of mushroom. Afterward, sauté up to the point when the liquids are discharged. Using pepper, as well as garlic powder, season them up to the point they become brilliant dark colored. This will be used in a short while.

5. Through medium-high setting, in a ten-inch skillet, include one more sprinkle of additional virgin olive oil as well as cauliflower. Afterward, using pepper, salt, and garlic powder, season and sauté them for around 240 to 300 seconds.

6. Through medium setting, in a ten-inch skillet, include spinach, mushrooms, and green onions. Keep this up for around half a minute, then include eggs into the mix. Pour the mixed ingredients above the cauliflower hash browns, then finish it with the salsa as well as mashed avocado.

Macros for this recipe are approximately:

- 725.3 in calories
- 26.77 g protein
- 40.72 g carbs
- 55.84 g fat
- 21.39 g fiber

Savory Sage and Cheddar Waffles

Servings: 12 waffles

Ingredients:

- one cup of Shredded Cheddar Cheese
- .5 tsp Salt
- one fourth teaspoon Garlic Powder
- two cup Coconut Milk
- .5 cup Water
- 3 tsp Baking Powder
- one tsp Sage
- 2 Eggs
- one and one third cup Coconut Flour
- three tablespoons of Coconut Oil

Instructions:

1. Heat your waffle iron you will need to do this in whatever directions from the manufacturer.
2. Mix the coconut flour, sage, garlic powder, salt, and baking powder in a mixing bowl.
3. Add liquid ingredients (water, oil, and milk). Afterward, mix them until the mixture thickens.
4. Include cheddar cheese.
5. Apply oil on the waffle cooker so as to avoid sticking later on. Afterward, pour one-third cup of the mixture to each mold, then put back the cover and let them cook under medium setting.

Macros for this recipe:

For each waffle

- 195.5 calories
- 17.47 g fats
- 3.49 net carbs
- 5.49 g protein
- 8.84 carbs
- 5.35 g fiber

Lunch

Lunch is where you need a pick me up and to get yourself going again. Here is a recipe for some amazing vegetarian collard green wraps. If you are looking for another culture to try your luck because this recipe is Greek. They have so many healthy vegetables in this recipe, which is amazing, but there is also a recipe for a great sauce to add some extra flavor to the wraps—and as long as you watch your intake, your calories should be alright as well.

Vegetarian Greek Collard Wraps

Lunch is where you need a pick me up and to get yourself going again. Here is a recipe for some amazing vegetarian collard green wraps. If you are looking for another culture to try your luck because this recipe is Greek. They have so many healthy vegetables in this recipe, which is amazing, but there is also a recipe for a great sauce to add some extra flavor to the wraps and as long as you watch your intake, your calories should be alright as well.

The recipe makes four servings and the directions are as follows.

Tzatziki Sauce

- two tbsp. minced fresh dill
- one tsp garlic powder
- two tbsp. olive oil
- two point five ounces of cucumber, seeded and grated (¼-whole)
- one tbsp. white vinegar
- One cup full-fat plain Greek yogurt
- Salt and pepper to taste

The Wrap

- four large cherry tomatoes – halved
- half a block feta, cut into four (one-inch thick) strips (four-oz.)
- four large collard green leaves – washed
- one medium cucumber, julienned
- half a cup purple onion, diced
- eight whole Kalamata olives – halved
- half a medium red bell pepper, also julienned

85

Instructions:

1. For the sauce, put the ingredients in a container and mix them until the desired texture is achieved, then put them in the fridge to cool. Don't forget to extract the liquids from the cucumbers.

2. Upon cleaning the leaves thoroughly, cut the stems from every single one of them.

3. Pour about 2 tbsp. of sauce on the wraps, then evenly flatten them.

4. Place onion, feta, pepper, tomatoes, cucumber, and olives on each wrap. Make sure that they are coupled in such a way that they would not easily get untangled from one another, as it would be quite messy if otherwise. Remember—the presentation is as important as the taste, and this is no exception.

5. Fold as you would a burrito.

6. Slice each wrap into two, then prepare for consumption.

Macros

- 165.4 calories
- 7.36 g net carbs
- 11.25 g fat
- 6.98 g protein

Snacks

Snacks are an important staple in any diet as well because if you feel deprived and restricted this diet will make you unhappy and that's one of the things that many people say that they feel on diets and you do not want that because you tend to slip or give yourself really unhealthy meals when you begin to feel like you are not getting the food your body is wanting.

Pimento Cheese

This is a really delicious recipe for a pimento cheese that works really well for a dipping sauce or that you can eat straight away depending on your preferences. I personally think it goes really well with some healthy vegetables.

Ingredients:

- Chopped fresh chives or fresh parsley, for decoration to add to the dish
- 4 tbsp. pickled jalapeños, finely chopped
- 1 tbsp. Dijon mustard
- 1 tsp paprika powder
- 5⅓ tbsp. mayonnaise
- 1 pinch cayenne pepper
- 4 oz. shredded cheddar cheese

Instructions:

1. Mix all the ingredients together, leave out the chives for the moment.

2. Let it chill in your fridge for at least an hour, for this recipe preferably two.

3. Form them into balls or place onto serving spoons.

4. Decorate with the chives that you had set aside before.

5. This recipe will yield about four servings for you and can actually keep for around five days in the refrigerator, which is awesome because you will have it for a few days!

Macros

- 765.1 calories

- 73.4 g fat

- 8.6 g carb

- 15.3 g protein

Roasted Asparagus with Easy Blender Hollandaise Sauce

The Hollandaise sauce takes this roasted asparagus dish over the top.

- Prep Time will be 10 minutes.
- Cook Time will be 10 minutes.
- Total Time will be 20 minutes.

Servings: 4

Calories: 296kcal

Ingredients:
- One lb. asparagus
- Juice of half a lemon or more to taste. This will depend on your preference
- cayenne pepper to taste, once again it will depend on your preferences
- three egg yolks
- one tbsp. grass-fed ghee or butter melted
- salt & pepper to taste
- butter heated

Instructions:

1. Preheat your oven to 425 degrees.

2. Toss asparagus with one tbsp. of the butter ,salt, and pepper—and roast until it starts to caramelize but make sure that it is still crisp (about 10 minutes).

3. Add in your egg yolks, lemon juice, and cayenne pepper to a blender and blend a few seconds until combined. With blender running, pour the hot ghee or butter whichever you chose, into the blender in slow steam until combined. Taste and add more lemon juice, cayenne pepper, and salt if needed. Everyone's taste buds are different some may add more some may leave it as is. Thin with a little warm water if you so desire.

4. Drizzle your sauce over the asparagus and serve the remaining sauce on the side

Macros

- 296 calories

- 4 g carbs

- 4 g protein

- 29 g fat

- 17 g saturated fat

As you can see, this recipe is low in carbs but it is high in other things you need like iron and potassium. It also has some protein and other vitamins that you need to make sure that you have enough of. If you have noticed your lacking in some of these areas, a recipe like this might be able to get you back to where you need to be.

You can also make plates of vegetables for a good snack and that will add some much-needed vegetables to your day. Remember that with a vegetarian diet you need to get enough. The healthy snacks will be super helpful here as well because you'll be getting them and have a yummy snack.

You could make a plate of broccoli and cheese. Or hardboiled eggs and some nuts. You can make all sorts of different combinations to make yourself feel full and make sure you are following your diet wisely. The best way to go about this is knowing what foods complement each other the best and what foods work well for you and each other. Finding the foods that will help your diet is really going to make it a lot easier on you when you are planning meals and snacks.

Dinner

Dinner is where we normally eat our most calories, or we eat our biggest meal. Now in some cultures, this is not true, and they actually eat lunch as their biggest meal or shift the meals around so that they do not really have a big meal throughout the day. Which is good as well every culture has different things that we can learn from, and all the information is good to look into. You might decide that you like having dinner at lunchtime or if you are a busy on the go type person you might prefer to have lots of small meals during the day instead of a big one. Either way you choose is fine as everyone has different wants and needs and every person's goals are different as well. If dinner is where you get your calories and find that this is where you eat the most, there are some great recipes for that—and if you want a light dinner, there are just as many good meals and recipes for that as well. The key is to do your research and find the recipes you like or want to try.

A really nice recipe I found for a different take on a classic is instead of grilled cheese we have found a recipe for zucchini grilled cheese. This is a very tasty unique twist on a classic dish, and it is a good way to get some more vegetables in your meal.

Zucchini Grilled Cheese Sandwich

Servings: 3-4

Ingredients:

- Vegetable oil, for cooking the dish
- Two cups of grated zucchini
- one large egg
- Two cups of shredded Cheddar cheese
- half a cup of freshly grated Parmesan
- two green onions, thinly sliced
- one-fourth of a cup of cornstarch

Instructions:

1. Squeeze all of the excess moisture out of your zucchini with a clean kitchen towel. Anything sticking to the towel will get onto your food. In a medium bowl, combine your zucchini with the egg, Parmesan cheese, green onions, and your cornstarch.

2. In a large skillet, pour enough vegetable oil to layer the bottom of the pan. Scoop about one-fourth of your cup of the zucchini mixture onto one side of the pan and shape into a small square. Repeat this process to form another patty on the other side of your skillet.

3. Cook until lightly golden on both sides of the patty, it is going to be about 4 minutes per side. Remove from heat to drain them on

paper towels and repeat with remaining zucchini mixture. Wipe skillet clean afterward.

4. Place two zucchini patties in the same skillet you just cleaned over medium heat. Top both with the shredded cheese, then place two more zucchini patties on top to form two sandwiches. Cook until the cheddar cheese has melted, this process will be about 2 minutes per side.

5. Repeat with all of your remaining ingredients. Serve immediately.

Macros for this recipe approximate at:

- 1,388.6 calories

- 109.7 g fat

- 28.6 g carbs

- 77.7 g protein

Cauliflower fried rice

- One fourth a cup of onions
- One fourth a teaspoon of salt
- Finely chopped garlic cloves four of them
- One tablespoon of ginger minced
- Half a cup of chopped bell pepper
- One cup of peas and carrots
- One teaspoon of sesame oil that's toasted
- One to two teaspoons of Asian chili sauce
- One teaspoon of soy sauce. If you can find low sodium soy sauce aim for that
- Half a head of medium cauliflower which equals between two and a half to three cups when you shred it
- One fourth a head of broccoli which is about one cup shredded or you can use more cauliflower
- Dash of black pepper. Be generous or to your own taste

Directions:

Cook both the onion and the garlic in oil over medium heat until the ingredients are golden.

Add your ginger, and vegetables besides the broccoli and cauliflower to your dish and add salt. Then mix and cover the dish before cooking it for three to four minutes.

Add your cauliflower and broccoli, sauces and

seasonings together. If you need them more fine, use a processor.

Cover and cook the dish for five minutes. Fluff the ingredients really well before you cover again and let sit to steam for another two minutes. You want the cauliflower to be cooked to a texture that is a little more than what al dente is but not enough that it loses its bite.

Taste and fluff again. Serve hot.

Macros are as follows.

- 106 calories
- 3 g in total fat
- 632 mg sodium
- 606 mg potassium
- 17 g total carbs
- 5 g protein
- 5 g dietary fiber
- 144.2% vitamin C
- 108% vitamin A

Recipes are so helpful when you are trying to eat healthier and change your life and how you think about your meals. Great informational sites out there will be so good to help with this, but we've taken the initiative to find some for you.

Vegetarian Keto Meal Ideas

Breakfasts Ideas

- Vegetables and eggs with avocado fried in coconut or olive oil
- Eggs frittata with asparagus and avocado
- Vegetable and feta omelet fried in coconut or olive oil
- Smoothie made from coconut cream, some berries, ice, full-fat yogurt, almond butter, and stevia extract

Lunch Ideas

- Egg and avocado salad
- Mixed greens salad with avocado, mozzarella, pesto, olives, bell pepper, onions, a few nuts, lemon juice, and extra virgin olive oil dressing
- Vegetarian low-carb Greek salad with feta, tomatoes, onions, olives, fresh Greek spices, and extra virgin olive oil
- Stir-fried cauliflower "rice" with veggies and eggs

Dinner Ideas

- Cheese pizza with cauliflower crust and broccoli
- Pasta made with zucchini noodles and Keto alfredo sauce
- Portobello "steak" with kale salad and cauliflower mashed potatoes
- Eggplant parmesan fried in coconut oil

Seven-Day Plan

This seven-day plan can also help. It includes breakfast, lunch, dinner, dessert and a snack. It can show you that this diet has a lot of variety and you are not just stuck with one type of food. You can enjoy just as many dishes on a Vegetarian Ketogenic diet as you can on a meat eater's diet.

Day one

- Meal one – A smoothie made with strawberries and tofu on the side.
- Meal two – Greek collard wraps
- Smaller meal or snack – Cucumber Slices paired with Olive Tapenade.
- Meal three – Zucchini grilled cheese sandwiches.
- Sweet treat – Almond Crust with Red grape truffles.

Day two

- Meal one – Fruit with high fiber content cereals. This is going to help you hit those numbers we mentioned.
- Meal two – Summer Vegetable Bisque accompanied with a Soy Egg Salad.
- Smaller meal or snack – Vegetable Spring Rolls with a Spicy Peanut Sauce for extra flavor.
- Meal three – Spinach Pie with a Vegetable Salad.
- Sweet treat – Chocolate Silk Pie.

Day three

- Meal one – Scrambled Tofu. This starts off with some protein.
- Meal two – Zucchini noodles and avocado sauce.
- Smaller meal or snack – Spinach and Artichoke Dip. This is a savory and delicious snack.
- Meal three – Vegetarian Sloppy Joes with a Green Vegetable Salad.
- Sweet treat – Blueberry Soy Cheesecake.

Day four

- Meal one – Protein shake along with fruit may be an old classic but it is healthy for this meal plan.
- Meal two – Tofu with Vegetable Chef Salad.
- Smaller meal or snack – Jalapeno Hummus with Jicama Sticks a spicy but yummy treat.
- Meal three – Spinach Pesto along with Roasted Eggplant Lasagna.
- Sweet treat – Apple Crumb Pie.

Day five

- Meal one – Tofu Benedict. A good thing to remember is tofu takes on the flavor of whatever sauce or marinade you will be using in this dish.
- Meal two – Vegetable Slaw with spiced lentil soup (you might want to sub out the lentils; remember that there is carb bomb, and you do not need a carbohydrate bomb with this diet).
- Smaller meal or snack – Eggplant Dip along with Whole Grain Crackers.
- Meal three – Parsley with Portobello Patties.
- Sweet treat – Poached Pears in Chocolate Sauce.

Day six

- Meal one – Coffee with Chocolate Smoothie (coffee done right is okay for ketogenic).
- Meal two – Spiced Tempeh with a Vegetable Salad.
- Smaller meal or snack – Mushrooms stuffed with delicious Pine Nuts. (If your high in carbs already you can sub for a better nut)
- Meal three – Sesame-Stuffed Portobello Mushrooms
- Sweet treat – Fudge Truffles for a sweet end to your day.

Day seven

- Meal one – Mushroom Frittata with Spinach this will start your day with vitamins.
- Meal two – Four Hearts Salad Serve with Split Pea Soup with Cabbage.
- Smaller meal or snack–Celery stuffed with hummus this makes a filling snack that's perfect for staying in your goals.
- Meal three – Stuffed Eggplant with Vegetable salad were getting more greens in your system for those vitamins you need.
- Sweet treat – Apple and Zucchini Cake, which is a clever way to get in more veggies.

Now, with this list, we are seeing the meat being replaced with the alternatives made from soy. This is what a lot of vegetarians do and that's fine, but just remember to monitor your soy intake closely as it may cause unpleasant side effects.

Desserts

For some added bonus here are some really delicious dessert recipes. One added pleasure of this diet is that you can have dessert, but you need to remember to stay healthy. This recipe for amazing brownies is an amazing way to sneak in some extra vegetables into your last meal of the day.

Zucchini Brownies

Servings: 20~24 brownies

Ingredients:

- Half a cup shredded zucchini (100g)
- One-third of a cup of applesauce, or yogurt such as coconut milk yogurt. If you are needing more protein at the end of your day you can use Greek yogurt instead of coconut milk but that will alter the nutrition value of the recipe if you make substitutions
- one cup plus two additional tablespoons of water
- two teaspoons of pure vanilla extract
- Three tablespoons of flax meal
- Half a cup and two additional tablespoons of vegetable or coconut oil
- Three fourths a cup of cocoa powder
- One cup coconut flour
- A half a teaspoon of salt
- A half a teaspoon of baking soda
- Three fourths a cup of sugar, or xylitol if you are wanting to go a for sugar-free option
- One-sixteenth of a teaspoon of uncut stevia, or two extra tablespoons of sugar
- A half a cup of mini chocolate chips, optional depending on preference and taste

Instructions:

1. You will need to preheat your oven to 350F and line a 9×13 baking dish with parchment paper. Then set aside for later.

2. In a large mixing bowl, whisk together the first six of your ingredients on the list and let sit at least for five minutes. (Tip: Shred zucchini in a food processor if you have one or can get access to one for fine shreds.)

3. Combine all other ingredients in a separate bowl and stir very well.

4. Pour wet into dry, and then stir until evenly mixed.

5. After everything is evenly mixed you will then pour into the baking dish.

6. Using a full sheet of parchment or wax paper, press down very firmly until the brownie batter evenly covers the pan.

7. Bake nineteen to twenty minutes, then pat down hard with a pancake spatula or another sheet of parchment. (If the recipe is still undercooked, it is fine. Just put them in your fridge overnight and they'll firm up!)

8. Let zucchini brownies sit at least fifteen minutes before trying to cut into squares—and if at all possible, wait until the next day to

consume them. If you wait, they will have twice as much flavor as if you did not.

9. An additional tip: as a general rule, cutting brownies with a plastic knife prevents crumbling. This will make twenty to twenty-four squares—plenty for one person or family members and friends if you feel willing to share.

For extra sweetness, you can frost your brownies with this recipe.

Ingredients:

- Half a cup of cocoa powder
- Two tablespoons of pure maple syrup or agave
- One half a cup of virgin coconut oil, melted

Instructions:

1. Mix all of your frosting ingredients together to form a sauce.

2. Spread sauce over the zucchini brownies, then place in the fridge or freeze if you would like for ten to twenty minutes.

3. The sauce will then transform itself into a delicious fudgy chocolate frosting that makes a perfect added sweetness to this dish.

4. These brownies taste much richer if you are patient enough to wait until the next day—after the flavors have had a chance to intensify.

5. Due to the melty nature of the frosting, these frosted brownies will do best if they are stored in your fridge or freezer. They will thaw very well.

Macros for this recipe are per brownie.

- 83 calories

- 6.2 g total fat

- 6.8 g total carbs

- 3 g dietary fiber

- 1.4 g protein

Chocolate Brownie Cheesecake

Servings: 1 cheesecake

Brownie

Ingredients:

- one cup plus two additional tablespoons of your milk of choice (side note: milk is high in both sugar and carbs, two things that are a no go on your diet. For this recipe, I would recommend finding alternative milk. There are a few soy milk types that offer fewer carbs than regular.
- half a cup and two additional tablespoons of oil
- one tablespoon of pure vanilla extract
- one cup spelled or white flour, or packed three fourths a cup Bob's GF
- one cup cocoa powder (I used mostly regular, plus two tablespoons of Dutch, to make one cup)
- one fourth a teaspoon plus one eighth a teaspoon of salt
- one-half teaspoon of baking powder
- one half of a cup of brown sugar or packed one half of a cup of coconut sugar
- one third a cup of unrefined sugar OR stevia baking blend (side note: too many artificial sweeteners are bad for this diet as well as too much sugar will also affect your numbers and

percentages. Make sure your keeping track of the amount you're taking in because it is important to stay on track. You will notice many vegan desserts and ketogenic desserts use artificial sweeteners in their desserts, so this is a good tip to remember)

- two tablespoons of flax meal or cornstarch, optional
- half a cup of mini chocolate chips, optional (depends on preference and taste)

Instructions:

1. Whisk together the first 3 ingredients on this list, then set aside for later.

2. Preheat your oven to 350F.

3. Grease a 9-inch springform pan and then set aside for later.

4. In a large mixing bowl, thoroughly combine all remaining ingredients.

5. Pour wet into dry and stir to combine, then pour into your prepared pan.

6. Smooth down and make even. Bake for twelve minutes.

Cheesecake

- twenty-four ounces of cream cheese, a good recommendation would be as to nondairy
- two cups plain yogurt, such as coconut milk yogurt (if your needing protein you can sub for Greek yogurt just know it will alter your nutrition on this recipe)
- two and one-half teaspoons of pure vanilla extract
- one half of a cup of sugar or maple syrup, honey, or xylitol for a sugar-free option if you are trying to eliminate sugar from your new diet as well
- three fourths a cup of cocoa powder (I used mostly regular, plus two tablespoons of Dutch, to make up the full amount)

Instructions:

1. Preheat your oven to 350 F.

2. Then, proceed to fill a 9×13 pan about halfway with water, and place it on your oven's lower rack.

3. Bring cream cheese to room temperature next.

4. In a blender or food processor, beat all cheesecake ingredients just until smooth. (Make sure that on this step you do not overbeat—if you overbeat, you will be introducing air bubbles that could burst while

there in the oven and thus cause cracking in your cheesecake.)

5. Smooth into the 9-inch springform pan with the baked brownies.

6. Place on the middle rack above the other pan.

7. Bake for thirty minutes, and do not open the oven during this time.

8. When the time is up, you need to leave the oven door closed and turn off heat.

9. You need to leave in the closed oven for an additional five minutes.

10. Then, you may remove—it will look underdone—and let cool for twenty minutes before placing the still-underdone cheesecake in the fridge.

11. Chill for at least 6 hours, during which time it will firm up.

Macros for this recipe are the following.

- 231 calories
- 16.4 g total fat
- 3.6 g dietary fiber
- 3.4 g protein
- 22.1 g total carbs
- 6.5 saturated fat

Vegan Coconut Macaroons

If you are a fan of coconut, and the flavor it brings to dishes and desserts then you'll love these macaroons. Macaroons are gaining popularity in the United States and other countries around the world, so this would be a great recipe to share with friends or family. Or even make them for a party.

Servings: 24 macaroons

These macarons are dipped in a dark chocolate, and they are full of the healthy fats you need as a ketogenic and sweetened with monk fruit—essentially a perfect fat bomb for Keto—but as stated above, Keto bombs are not the way to go for this diet, and you should sustain yourself with other foods instead because these do not really do anything for you. We have included one in this book, however, to show you what one looks like.

Ingredients:

- two-and-a-half cups of unsweetened shredded coconut, divided
- half a cup of almond flour
- half a cup of monk fruit sweetener (or sweetener of choice) remember not to use too many sweeteners in dessert recipes
- one-half a cup of aquafaba
- one teaspoon of vanilla extract
- one-half a teaspoon of almond extract
- pinch of salt

- one-half cup of vegan dark chocolate, melted (for dipping) if this is your preference

Instructions:

1. Preheat your oven to 350F and line a baking dish with parchment paper or silicone mat.

2. Take one cup of coconut and place it in the oven for eight to ten minutes.

3. Add all of your ingredients to a large bowl including the toasted coconut and mix it up well.

4. Take tablespoon round cookie scoops and place on baking sheet as well.

5. Bake for eighteen to twenty minutes.

6. Melt half a cup of the vegan dark chocolate for the dipping sauce. When cookies are cool to touch, you can dip the bottoms in and place them on parchment paper and put in the fridge to set for five to ten minutes. If you are not dipping them in the chocolate, they do not need to be refrigerated at all and you can eat them sooner.

7. Serve with your favorite nondairy milk and enjoy!

Macros for this recipe are approximated at:

- 2402.4 in calories

- 168.35 g fat

- 132.65 g carbs

- 32.5 g protein

As a side note to this recipe, it is worth noticing that they said nondairy milk. Milk is bad for Ketogenic people, so you will need to find a substitute that suits your diet. Almond milk is usually a good idea.

Vegan Keto Peanut Butter Chocolate Pumpkins

These tasty treats are a perfect addition to any meal. Another bonus is that these are totally vegan so you are not hurting animals at all by making this, which is better for you and the planet. The time on this is a bit long though so be sure that you have time carved out for this as it will take three hours and thirty minutes.

Servings: 10 pumpkins

Many ketogenic diets are about cutting out sugar, so this Keto fat bomb is a good recipe for people who do not want sugar in their desserts. Remember, though, that fat bombs are not considered healthy and that they are unnecessary. If you have to use them, do not rely on them alone.

Ingredients:

- liquid stevia, to taste (optional), depends on your preference and tastes
- two tablespoons of MCT oil
- one teaspoon vanilla extract
- One-fourth of a cup of coconut milk_powder, divided
- one-fourth of a cup cocoa butter
- One-fourth of a cup of unsweetened peanut butter
- One tablespoon of chia seeds
- Instructions you will need for this recipe

Instructions:

1. In a small mixing bowl, you will need to begin to stir together two tablespoons of the coconut milk powder with the peanut butter along with the chia seeds, then you will mix in stevia (if you are using one).

2. The "dough" should be firm enough to roll into little balls. If it is not, you will need to chill it in the fridge until it is! You will not be able to use them the same way that is needed if you do not.

3. Roll the dough into ten balls, you need to make sure they are equal in size and then flatten them, so they form discs. Mine were a bit more than one-half tablespoons of each and measured around an inch in diameter or two point five centimeters and were about ten centimeters tall

4. Chill these for twenty minutes until they are totally firm. They need to be totally firm.

5. Using your preferred method (I tend to go with a double boiler setup), to melt together your oils. When they are completely melted, you will need to stir in two tablespoons of the coconut milk powder and the vanilla extract. Then Stir until they are combined.

6. In your silicon mold of choice. Obviously, I went with the pumpkin molds because of Halloween. Pour in around one teaspoon of the cocoa butter mixture into each of the ten spots on the mold. You want just enough to cover the bottom evenly.

7. Freeze the partially-filled mold until the small amount of cocoa butter mixture is totally chilled. This works well because This should be around the same time that the peanut butter discs harden to where they need to be.

8. Remove everything from your freezer and place one peanut butter disc into each spot on your mold, on top of the cocoa butter layer.

9. Stir the remaining cocoa butter mixture so it recombines, then distribute it evenly over the peanut butter discs. If it does not cover everything just make sure you got the sides.

10. Let it cool around 180 additional minutes up to the point that everything has hardened fully.

Finally, if you found this book useful in any way, a review on Amazon is always appreciate

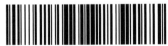

Made in the USA
Middletown, DE
16 March 2019